RETHINKING DRINKING AND SPORT

Rethinking Drinking and Sport
New Approaches to Sport and Alcohol

CATHERINE PALMER
University of Tasmania, Australia

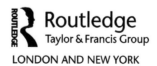

Routledge
Taylor & Francis Group

LONDON AND NEW YORK

First published 2015 by Ashgate Publishing

2 Park Square, Milton Park, Abingdon, Oxfordshire OX14 4RN
52 Vanderbilt Avenue, New York, NY 10017

Routledge is an imprint of the Taylor & Francis Group, an informa business

First issued in paperback 2020

British Library Cataloguing in Publication Data
A catalogue record for this book is available from the British Library

The Library of Congress has cataloged the printed edition as follows:
Palmer, Catherine (Sociologist)
   Rethinking drinking and sport : new approaches to sport and alcohol / by Catherine Palmer.
      pages cm
   Includes bibliographical references and index.
   ISBN 978-1-4094-5337-6 (hardback)
   1. Drinking of alcoholic beverages. 2. Athletes. I. Title.

HV5020.P355 2015
362.292088'796–dc23

                                                                            2015011045

ISBN 978-1-4094-5337-6 (hbk)
ISBN 978-0-367-59803-7 (pbk)

Contents

List of Figures

Abbreviations and Acronyms

AFL	Australian Football League
AMO	Alcohol Management Operation
ANPAA	Association Nationale en Alcoologie et Addictologie
BRIC	Brazil, Russia, India and China
FIFA	Fédération Internationale de Football Association
GSP	Good Sports programme
IOC	International Olympic Committee
SANFL	South Australian National Football League
SBI	Sports-based interventions
TAC	Transport Accident Commission
UKCAPP	UK Community Alcohol Prevention Programme

Acknowledgements

The writing of this book has benefited from much intellectual sparring with friends and colleagues at conferences, in corridors and pubs. I thank Martin Roderick, Jim McKay and Kim Toffoletti for their helpful comments on early drafts of work that have subsequently been included here. Larry Wenner and the *International Review for the Sociology of Sport* provided an invaluable space for like-minded researchers to share their ideas and scholarship through the special issue on 'Sport and Alcohol'. Much of this work has helpfully shaped aspects of my own.

Di Heckenberg provided superb and timely research assistance, and the University of Tasmania some welcome support for the project. Thank you all.

To David, of course, and Wilkie, for the distractions.

Finally, thank you to Neil Jordan at Ashgate for supporting the project and seeing it develop from a pony to a pint.

Preface

The idea for this book was prompted by what I saw to be a gap in social science approaches to sport-related drinking. Almost without exception, sport is perceived as being either awash with alcohol – a handmaiden to alcohol industry sponsorship – or a site where the conduct of professional male athletes when drunk (typically, but not exclusively, across the various football codes) is subject to much media and moral scrutiny in the countries where these codes dominate the sporting landscape. In short, sport-related drinking is most typically cast as a male pursuit where drinking practices are theorised through the lens of 'hegemonic masculinity' (Connell, 1987; 1995; Connell and Messerschmidt, 2005).

While not disputing that these issues exist, my starting point for this book is that there is considerably more to the 'sport-alcohol nexus' (Palmer, 2011) than just assumptions of normative gendered behaviour. There is already a wealth of literature devoted to examining sport and masculinity, and masculinity and alcohol, and it is not my intention to add significantly to that body of research. Instead, the book offers a series of case studies and analyses of sport-related drinking that seek to complement and extend the literature on sport-related drinking and masculinity. As I elaborate in the ensuing chapters, the assumptions and orientations inherent in such framings of sport run the risk of obscuring or missing entirely different relationships between sport and alcohol, as well as other theoretical frameworks through which sport-related drinking might be explained, interpreted or analysed. It is these ways of rethinking drinking that the book is more centrally concerned with. In other words, it is the kind of issues and relationships between sport and alcohol that *haven't* been written about that strike me as being fairly significant oversights when attempting to advance a richer understanding of sport-related drinking, and it is these that are explored in the following pages.

The kinds of questions and relationships between sport and alcohol that orient the book include: how do non-drinking fans and athletes (both men and women) construct and negotiate their identity in an environment where strong normative codes of drinking exist? What about men who embody different forms of masculine identities such as older men, gay athletes and fans, or men who reside outside of the major metropoles of North America, Australia and the United Kingdom; in the Global South, for example? What about female drinking in sport? Do women involved in sport 'do drinking' in the ways we now associate with (white, heterosexual) men? Does 'hegemonic masculinity' still have analytical utility when women are the subjects of study? What of drinking practices among non-traditional sports, and individual rather than team sports? What roles do religion and ethnicity play in people's understandings, experiences and articulations of sport-related drinking? In what ways does class and socio-economic advantage or disadvantage interact with the sport-alcohol nexus? Issues of inclusion and exclusion are at the heart of the cultural politics of sport-related drinking, yet have not been fully articulated. How does 'place' and where people live and drink influence drinking as it relates to sport? Certainly, the spatial dimensions of the night-time economy, where a range of leisure pursuits including drinking are concentrated around particular streets and sites in urban centres, have been noted, yet these analyses have not been fully extended to discussions of sport-related drinking. These were the kinds of questions and observations I began to ask of my own research, prompted in part by the largely stereotypical framings of drinking, men and sport I alluded to earlier.

My concern in the next nine chapters then is to not simply reproduce what we know already about sport-related drinking but to reassess and reinvigorate the theoretical frameworks and dominant orthodoxies so as to better approach the complex and at times contradictory range of social actors and drinking practices within the sport-alcohol nexus. Studies of sport and alcohol provide valuable insights into understanding the complexities of social relations in late modernity, and the role that one or both can – and have – played in reconfiguring individual and collective identities, and this is the abiding interest of the book.

Anthropologists, sociologists and geographers, among others, have been acutely alert to the sociality, commensality and spatiality of shared drinking in other empirical contexts, including office Christmas parties, Hen and Stag nights, backpacker tours, shore leave, university 'Fresher' weeks, and school breaks, as well as the more traditional anthropological studies of ritualised drinking associated with various rites of passage, yet the social meanings that are shared and carried through drinking as it occurs in *sporting* contexts have been largely overlooked in these fine-grained ethnographic analysis of drinking. While social anthropologists, in particular, have long had an interest in how, what, where and why people drink, and the meanings that are carried through drinking rituals and drinking transactions, *sport-related* drinking has, as a rule, tended to elude sustained ethnographic scrutiny. Extending the body of work on the social meanings and cultural practices that surround drinking through an ethnographically informed consideration of sports-associated drinking is a further focus of the book.

Related to this, one of the arguments I advance is that studies of sport-related drinking have tended to draw on a fairly limited repertoire of theoretical resources whereas social scientists with an interest in drinking more broadly have seen the possibilities of a broader range of theoretical frameworks for explaining the cultural practices, social interactions and, indeed, the consequences of consuming alcohol. That is, while academic interest in both sport and alcohol has expanded, far less has been written that explores the empirical *and* the theoretical connections between the activities. Drawing on these may lead to a more developed understanding of sport-related drinking, and one of the projects of the book is to develop a theoretically informed, empirically rich, understanding of sport-related drinking that takes us beyond popular orthodoxies and assumptions.

A third reason for the book is that the paradoxical and contradictory nature of the relationships between sport and alcohol has not yet been fully explored in a sustained and systematic way. Considerable attention has been paid – in media and popular discourse – to the 'problem' of sport-related drinking. Accounts of high profile sportsmen 'falling from grace' or being implicated in allegations of violence, sexual assault and other forms of abuse have captured our attention analytically, with excessive drinking, more often than not, occupying much of the space in critical research and scholarship. The particular rationalities that underpin the practices that encourage or condone these kinds of behaviours are addressed in the following pages, however part of the book's intellectual project is to move beyond the deficit model of conceptualising sport-related drinking as a 'problem'. Borrowing from Wilson (2005), I suggest that researchers should be able to discuss alcohol consumption from the perspective that it is not always a 'problem' but that, in some cases, it is both normal and normative.

The social contexts of the 'doing' of sport-related drinking in club, match or related settings are not the sole focus of the book. There is a growing number of sportsmen and women seeking treatment for alcohol and related problems (often following the kinds of public drinking incidents alluded to above), and this raises a series of questions concerning addiction, illness and recovery that may seem the antithesis to notions of role models, sporting identity, self-control, and sporting prowess more typically associated with high performing sportsmen and women. This emergent and under-explored relationship between sport and alcohol, its costs and consequences (i.e. suicide, relationship breakdowns, financial stresses, criminal and legal issues), as seen through the narratives and experiences of treatment and recovery by the athletes themselves are also explored as part of rethinking drinking and sport.

Finally, the flipside to these 'problems' of sport-related drinking is that sport (predominantly football and basketball) is frequently promoted as an intervention and an opportunity for recovery and rehabilitation programmes for many of the social problems associated with alcohol misuse. Notwithstanding the 'mythopoeic' (Coalter, 2007) nature of sport and the question of evidence as to whether such sports-based initiatives actually improve outcomes, the role of sport in prevention programmes for clients, usually young men, who are at risk of crime and violence through drug and alcohol misuse or who are seeking to recover and desist from drug and alcohol use also form part of the complex and contradictory discourse surrounding sport and alcohol when considered alongside the more visible accounts of 'the problem' of sport-related drinking, with its focus on the misdemeanours of high-profile sportsmen.

Drawing these threads together, it is an examination of the 'sport-alcohol nexus' (Palmer, 2011); that is, the interplay between sport and alcohol in terms of cultural practices and social identities, and, prevention, rehabilitation and culture change that is the focus of the next nine chapters.

Structure and Organisation

With this as background, the book is organised into two sections. The chapters in the first section – 'Social Practices and Drinking Identities' – explore a range of social practices and drinking identities associated with sport-related drinking. The first chapter introduces the key terms and definitions encountered in the rest of the book and offers an overview of the sport-alcohol nexus, the convergences and divergences between approaches from the health and social sciences, and some of the dominant themes and discourses that have dominated both academic and policy debates. Taking the over-reliance on the notion of hegemonic masculinity as its point of departure, the second chapter moves onto some of the alternative theoretical perspectives that can be used to understand, analyse and explain sport-related drinking. Working within a broad conceptual framework of 'contested leisure', the second chapter explores the work and creativity associated with sport-related drinking when it is conceived as 'calculated hedonism' (Szmigin, Griffin and Mistral, 2008) or as 'serious leisure' (Stebbins, 2001). In positioning sport-related drinking as a form of calculated hedonism – a framework adopted for studies of 'binge drinking' more broadly – the problem of pleasure is also introduced as a major barrier to uptake and compliance with a number of policies and strategies designed to minimise the harms and risks associated with sport-related drinking. In thinking about sport-related drinking as a form of 'serious leisure' due attention is paid to the creativity and emotional labour that often surrounds the activities of sporting groups and communities, including virtual ones, in which drinking plays a central part.

While the concern of the first two chapters is to re-think or re-theorise behaviours typically constructed as problematic in relation to sport and alcohol (such as binge drinking or male drinking), the last three chapters in this section then explore some of the new and emerging relationships between sport and alcohol. These chapters examine female drinkers, non-drinkers and the (auto)biographies of 'problem' drinkers that can shed light on particular relationships between sport and alcohol, as articulated and experienced by the individuals themselves. These are all under-explored and under-theorised groups and individuals in the sport-alcohol nexus, yet, in different ways, they raise a number of issues and concerns for the sociology of sport, leisure and consumption more broadly.

In essence, these chapters provide the empirical backdrop to the second half of the book – 'Tackling the Problem' – which focuses on the implications of these – and similar – behaviours for policy and practice. The chapters in this second section deal primarily with the relationships between sport, alcohol, prevention and rehabilitation, where sport provides a setting for a number of programmes aimed at the prevention of or recovery from alcohol-related abuses and, where rehabilitation settings can offer specialist treatment for sportsmen and women who struggle with alcohol and other addictions. Variously, the chapters i) examine and evaluate some of the strategies and initiatives that sporting clubs and communities have put in place to address, recognise, challenge and change the culture of drinking in sport; ii) address and critique particular interventions that use sport in prevention and rehabilitation programmes, and; iii) consider the broader implications raised in the book for health and social policy. Thus, the chapters on prevention and rehabilitation make important contributions to understanding sport and alcohol in a broader social context of drug and alcohol recovery, and wider debates about the night-time economy, law and order, health and welfare, and public policy.

The book refers to 'sport-related' drinking or 'sports-associated' drinking, and I use these terms fairly interchangeably. I've chosen these terms deliberately to capture the diversity of the behaviours and practices I am interested in. My intention is not to offer a definitive position on sport and alcohol, nor how the relationships involved should be approached theoretically, empirically or conceptually. Rather, it is to reinvigorate our understandings of the complex and at times contradictory range of drinkers and drinking practices within the sport-alcohol nexus.

While, the focus, in the main, is on the drinking practices enacted by sportsmen and women and sports fans, and their consequences, it is also, although less so, concerned with those affected by another's sport-related drinking. This relatively fluid understanding of the nature and extent of sports-related drinking highlights its problematic and paradoxical features, particularly in the context of industry promotion, health costs and consequences, regulation, governance and legislation, a discussion of which provides the broader social and policy backdrop to the book.

Two further qualifications are needed. Most of the work I refer to is written in English and is associated with or derived from the United Kingdom, United States or Australia as either a site for empirical investigation or as the place of origin of most investigators. There are, of course, researchers working, notably, in Northern Europe, South and Latin America, and Japan, but much of their work is inaccessible to the wider alcohol and drug research community, as it appears in documents with limited circulation either by language or region. Where this is the case, I direct the reader towards some of the conceptual linkages here. Equally, most of the empirical data I report is largely qualitative and socio-cultural in nature, which, in part, reflects my background and research interests as an interdisciplinary social scientist. Certainly, biological, biocultural and biophysical accounts of alcohol consumption, patterns and prevalence have been undertaken which can add value to socio-cultural studies, but, because I do not work in these fields, I refer to them somewhat tangentially.

My final disclaimer is that drug and alcohol policy, like other policy fields, moves fast and there will invariably be policy developments that will 'break' which I cannot describe in any real detail. Where possible, I've acknowledged this and suggested further research to accommodate these emerging policy agendas. Although alcohol and sport is the main focus of the book, other related behaviours such as gambling or recreational drug-taking are also addressed in the second half of the book, with its focus on policy, prevention and rehabilitation. As a research-informed, interdisciplinary social analysis of sport-related drinking, it is hoped that the book can make a unique contribution to the literature on sport and alcohol, its meanings, its associated problems, and its implications for theory, practice and policy.

PART I
Social Practices and Drinking Identities

Chapter 1
Mapping the Sport-Alcohol Nexus

This chapter:
- provides an overview of the sport-alcohol nexus and sets the context for the rest of the book;
- reviews the literature on drinking and drunkenness;
- examines the emerging issues for policy and practice in relation to sport-related drinking.

'No more booze for Bombers'

'Professional sports still failing in their duty of care when it comes to alcohol'

'Brendan Fervola's 13 hour bender and night of shame'

'Joey Barton gives up alcohol to save career'

'Sobriety rules at Rio'

Introduction

These quotes taken from Australian and British press coverage of sports stars and elite level competition provide the backdrop to much of what follows. Each reference details a different relationship to sport and alcohol. The mention of Brendan Fervola refers to the former Australian Rules footballer's drunken activities at the Brownlow Medal Count for *The Footy Show*, following an extended daytime drinking session in a popular Melbourne nightspot.[1] The claim that professional sport has failed in its duty-of-care follows the former Australian cricketer Andrew Symonds' admission to a series of alcohol-related problems. The 'Bombers giving up booze' reflects the policy of the Essendon football club abstaining from alcohol throughout the 2012 Australian Rules football season. The

---

1 Brendan Fervola is a former Australian Rules footballer who was stood down from his team and sacked from his job as a 'roving reporter' for *The Footy Show*, a popular television programme devoted to all things footy for urinating in public and groping a female guest at this football award's presentation evening.

Queens Park Rangers midfielder's decision to 'give up alcohol' refers to the six month stretch that Barton spent in prison for assault and affray after reportedly consuming ten pints and five bottles of lager in a single sitting, while the account of Gary Roberts being released by English football club Yeovil follows his journey through treatment and recovery for problems associated with alcohol misuse. The headline of 'sobriety at Rio' follows Kitty Chiller's – the Australian Olympic team Chef de Mission for the 2016 Games – call for a ban on alcohol in the Olympic Village and on the flight home. These brief snippets bring together some of the ways in which sport and alcohol intersect and alert us to just some of the contradictions and complexities of drinking and drinkers in sport with which this book is principally concerned.

The focus of the book is on what I've referred to elsewhere as the 'sport-alcohol nexus' (Palmer, 2011); that is, the myriad ways in which alcohol intersects with sport (see Figure 1.1).

The sport-alcohol nexus refers to the three-fold interplay between sport and alcohol in terms of:

  i.   cultural practices and social identities;
  ii. pleasurable and problematic relationships to alcohol, and,
  iii. prevention, rehabilitation and culture change.

Sport-related drinking can be understood, experienced and manifested as a set of social relationships, as a policy problem and as embedded in crucial narratives and practices of treatment and recovery.

Figure 1.1   The sport-alcohol nexus

Conceived as such, the sport-alcohol nexus is indeed a broad church. It includes a consideration and critique of sport-based drinking practices as they are popularly imagined primarily (and fairly crudely) as: i) male drinking that brings with it a host of concomitant health and social problems; ii) 'binge' and excessive alcohol consumption by players and fans; iii) promotional culture, such as alcohol sponsorship and advertising and, perhaps most importantly; iv) some of the counter-intuitive and under-explored relationships between sport and alcohol, such as women, non-drinkers and 'light' or social drinkers, as well as older men, gay men, non-Anglo men and other males who sit outside of normative assumptions of men in sport. Indeed, one of the central arguments developed in the book is that there is considerably more to sport-related drinking than what the media and popular discourse routinely presents.

The relative absence of discussion of drinking by female fans or sportswomen, the emergence of non-drinking sportsmen and women, the place or role of ethnicity and religion in shaping particular sport-related drinking practices, the intersection between drinking and locational disadvantage, shifting drinking patterns such as 'pre-loading' and domestic drinking that suggest a day-time as well as a night-time economy, and the growing visibility of 'athlete addicts', among other things, have all created a new set of research questions and problems for critical interrogation through sustained, theoretically informed, empirical social research. Taking forward this new research agenda in ways that challenge some of the existing orthodoxies and taken-for-granted positions in research, policy and practice is the intellectual project that lies at the heart of this book.

Adding to the complexity of the sport-alcohol nexus, a key feature of government policy in most Western neoliberal democracies is the use of sports-based interventions as a vehicle for social change in relation to alcohol misuse. In such programmes, sport is commonly promoted as a diversion to a range of health damaging, anti-social or criminal behaviour, where interventions provide opportunities for prevention and rehabilitation, particularly for marginalised and vulnerable population groups and for young people at risk of offending in urban areas. While the 'mythopoeic' (Coalter, 2007) nature of sport and its ability to adequately address complex social problems has been problematised in relation to this kind of community intervention and outreach work, sports-based alcohol intervention programmes continue to command considerable attention and scrutiny as to both their effectiveness and their potential to reproduce rather than redress structural inequalities. These debates are revisited in Chapter 7.

Equally, an increasing number of sportsmen and women are seeking treatment for alcohol-related problems, usually sparked by a misdemeanour or high profile fall from grace. Here, the pressures and demands of elite sport are positioned as the context or the environment within which substance misuse can occur. This too, is part of the sport-alcohol nexus and these issues are addressed in Chapter 5. Thus, the book considers the relationship between sport and alcohol as a contested and contradictory space for the expression of particular forms of identity through which a range of broader themes, questions and problematics can be interrogated and explored.

This three way consideration of sport as: i) a setting in which particular social identities can be constructed and reproduced through drinking-based practices; ii) the ways in which drinking is positioned as a 'problem' in sport, as well as; iii) some of the issues for prevention, treatment and recovery that are embedded in sport-related drinking requires some careful points of clarification and the rest of the chapter unfolds in the following way: I first map out the social and symbolic importance of drinking in sport and society more broadly. Here, key contributions to the sociality of drinking from disciplines such as sociology and social anthropology are explored. To complement this social science perspective on the social role of consuming alcohol, the chapter then reviews some of the positions from within the health and medical sciences. These are not meant to be viewed as opposing standpoints rather, ones that offer complementary, if at times contradictory perspectives on alcohol, sport and society more broadly.

What emerges from both perspectives however is the growing and continuing presence of drinking – sport-related or otherwise – in a number of policy debates more broadly, and the chapter then charts the key issues that underpin what is, at times, a contested and crowded policy agenda, where discourses of risk, regulation, governmentality, individual choice and agency, health and welfare, structure and social contexts frame a number of policy debates. From there, the chapter sketches out the key theoretical positions that have dominated studies of sport-related drinking and concludes with a note on data sources and the methodologies that will be employed in the more empirical chapters that follow.

But, a note on terminology is perhaps warranted first. Throughout the book, I use the terms 'the sport-alcohol nexus', 'sport-related drinking' and 'sports-associated drinking' fairly interchangeably. I've chosen these terms deliberately to capture the diversity and, to some extent the ambiguity of the behaviours and practices the book is concerned with. While, the focus, in the main, is on the drinking practices and their consequences as experienced, understood and enacted by sportsmen/women and by sports fans, it is also, although less so, concerned with those affected by another's sport-related drinking. At various stages, the book touches on some of the damage(s) done by another's sport-related drinking in a broader context of stigma, shame, violence, abuse, treatment and recovery.

Alcohol: An Introduction

Most Western democratic countries have a long history of drinking. Douglas (1987) notes that the modern use of alcohol has its cultural origins in rituals and religious belief systems, while early Mass Observation surveys in the United Kingdom suggest that drinking in public houses was an important form of social connection in the nineteenth and early twentieth centuries (Collins and Vamplew, 2002; Dimeo, 2013). Such traditions continue, and consuming alcohol is now synonymous with markers of both the memorable and the mundane, with births, weddings, deaths and other life occasions being celebrated or remembered through the consumption of alcohol. Drinking rituals are also used to define far less momentous passages, such as the daily or weekly transitions from work to leisure/ home, or even the beginning and completion of a specific task, where alcohol 'cues' the transition from work time to play time. As I elaborate shortly, the social dimensions of drinking have provided a rich source of data for social scientists across a range of disciplines and empirical and geographical contexts. Indeed, the perception of the 'value of alcohol for promoting relaxation and sociability' is one of the most significant generalisations to emerge from cross-cultural studies of drinking (Heath, 1995).

Alongside this interest in the social aspects of drinking, medical and health sciences began to look at the aetiology of alcohol consumption, and its effects on and consequences for individual and population health, where alcohol is widely considered to be a leading cause of preventable death, disease, injury and disability, contributing to 3.2 per cent of deaths and 4 per cent of disability adjusted life years globally (Casey, Harvey, et al., 2012). Bringing together a concern with the social aspects of drinking and the health costs and consequences of drinking, public policy in Northern and Western Europe, Northern America and Australasia, among others, developed an interest in drinking as a social problem, most notably 'binge' drinking, drinking by young people and drinking by young women where, with varying degrees of success, a range of policy responses to the 'problem' of drinking to excess have been formulated, such as the 'one punch' laws in New South Wales, Australia, introduced in early 2014 to punish offenders convicted of single blow hits resulting from street-based alcohol-fuelled violence.

Studies of sport-related drinking, I suggest, bring together many of the interests across the disciplinary paradigms of the social and health sciences and the concerns of public policy. As I explore in the chapters that follow, drinking in sporting contexts can be a source of enormous enjoyment and social connection among drinking peers, it is centrally located in debates about the health risks and consequences of alcohol consumption worldwide, and it is wholly constructed as a social problem that intersects with policy debates more broadly about access, affordability, regulation, governmentality, risk, individual choice, gender, age, urban space and the night-time economy.

Not surprisingly however, the epistemological and ontological assumptions that underpin these different disciplinary positions has meant that even fairly straightforward terms like 'alcohol', 'drinking' and 'drunkenness' can be used in quite different, if not contradictory ways. Although I posit a fairly crude distinction between the social sciences and the health or medical sciences, this is done for reasons of analytical simplicity. In practice, this separation is far too blunt. 'Alcohol studies' is a far more complex set of disciplinary interests and below is an attempt to synthesise rather than offer an exhaustive overview of the key themes and debates from the literature.

Alcohol in/and the Health Sciences

While the focus of the book, in the main, is on the social contexts of sport-related drinking, some preliminary comments on the place of alcohol in the health or medical sciences are worth briefly making. Alongside the social aspects of drinking, discussed shortly, the consumption of alcohol remains an abiding concern for the health and medical sciences. Research globally suggests that hazardous drinking is a serious social and public health problem (World Health Organization, 2011; Connor, et al., 2013). Focussing on just one country, Connor, et al. (2005) estimated that New Zealand suffered a net loss (i.e. after accounting for the hypothetical protective effects of alcohol consumption) of 11,900 years of life in the year 2000 and 26,000 disability-adjusted life years in 2002, due to alcohol consumption. Similar estimated statistics can be found for most other OECD countries as well.

The problem of drinking as a health issue and as a subject for health and medical science saw an increasing characterisation of alcohol and drug dependency as a disease or a pathological behaviour. It was soon realised however, that while a person may suffer the individual effects of alcohol misuse in terms of its physical effects on them, society as a whole suffers from the many consequences of alcohol abuse and dependence, and solutions to alcohol misuse became located within a public health model (Gilbert, 1993) whereby the endogenous, biological and 'agentic' aspects of alcohol and other drug use were emphasised when searching for treatment and solutions. Accordingly, ways of framing and attempting to understand alcohol use moved beyond a focus on the individual to a social or a population level focus on the consequences of alcohol and other drug use (Seddon, 2011).

It is this focus on the social aspects of drinking, the contexts in which it takes place, and the backgrounds and milieu that inform it, which frames much of the chapters that follow. That is, the book emphasises the notion that distinctive structural or cultural environments both frame and situate human behaviour, in this case sport-related drinking, and the diverse cultural practices that underpin and sustain it (Agar, 2003; Durrant and Thakker, 2003). In other words, while the 'problem' of drinking, particularly drinking to excess, remains a key concern for health professionals, my interest here is less with the health-damaging behaviour and the consequences of drinking, and more with the social dimensions and understandings that underpin it. As mentioned previously, a key aim of the book is to move beyond the deficit model of conceptualising sport-related drinking as a 'problem'. Borrowing from Wilson (2005), I suggest that researchers should be able to discuss alcohol consumption and conduct research into alcohol consumption from the perspective that it is not always a problem, but in some cases, it is both normal and normative, and a rich source of pleasure, enjoyment and sociality.

Understanding the normal and normative dimensions of alcohol consumption may, in turn, influence behaviour change and public health or policy interventions. Writing about drinking and young people in Europe, Eisnebach-Stangl and Thom note 'to understand youthful binge drinking and associated behaviours, and to find ways of intervening to prevent or reduce harm, it is necessary to understand the prevailing concept(s) of acceptable and unacceptable forms of intoxication and intoxicated behaviours and its/their wider social and cultural determinants' (2009: 1). While Schwandt offers the caveat that 'context is never at once and completely capable of articulation' (2001: 36); structure and agency work in concert, macro institutions exert force over micro or individual settings or locales (gender or class, for example, generates social and contextual effects in many locales all at once); the notion of the social rather than the individual, the contextual rather than the pathological is the lens through which much of the book is framed.

Alcohol in/and the Social Sciences

Even a cursory scan of leading social science journals indicates that issues of alcohol use and misuse are increasingly subject to critical scrutiny from scholars across a number of disciplines. The spatial aspects of drinking and drunkenness, for example, receive attention from human and cultural geographers. Anthropologists have described the social nature of drinking. Shifting patterns of drinking towards what is seen as a 'culture of intoxication', particularly among young people, have been documented by those in sociology, criminology and policy studies, and the visual and representational aspects of advertising and sponsorship have been considered by consumer behaviourists and proponents of Cultural Studies alike. While much of this literature is examined in more detail in ensuing chapters, my focus for the moment is on the social nature of drinking, for this provides a key point of departure to understanding sport-related drinking as an 'everyday', normal and normative cultural practice among sportsmen and women, and sports consumers, fans and supporters. The analyses of these can then be applied to social and public policy and particular interventions as they relate to prevention, treatment and recovery, which are examined in the second half of the book.

The sociality of drinking
At the risk of privileging a particular disciplinary perspective, Social Anthropology has made a significant contribution to advancing our understandings of the 'everyday' social and cultural aspects of alcohol consumption (see Douglas, 1987; Heath, 2000; De Garine and de Garine, 2002; Moore, 1990; 1992; McDonald, 1994; Wilson, 2005). Hunt and Barker (2001) summarise the field, situating anthropological studies of drinking within both a wider context of anthropological thought and research as well as the 'wider social and political context that takes account of the organizational, funding and conceptual influences, constraints and pressures that operate on anthropologists who wish to conduct research on alcohol and drug issues' (2001: 165).

The cross-cultural aspects of social anthropology have been particularly useful for understanding patterns and convergences in drinking practices and behaviours. As Room notes 'comparative cross-cultural studies offer particular opportunities to deepen our understanding of causal and interactional patterns among the factors under study' (1996: 228). The idea of drunkenness as an aspect of hegemonic masculinity in 'laddish' cultures, for example, would be 'strongly opposed by the men of rural Spain in the late 1970s', where 'intoxication was ugly and socially disapproved of' (Clayton and Harris, 2008: 313), and it is the tensions and contradictions inherent in studies of drinking, sport-related or otherwise, that this book is principally concerned with.

What is drunk, by whom, under what conditions and to what ends, are questions that remain fundamental to the project of Social Anthropology. Beccaria and Sande (2003), for example, in their comparative study of drinking games by young people in Norway and Italy, note that drinking cultures and practices across what they term 'wet' and 'dry' settings are becoming increasingly similar. For young people in both Italy and Norway, drinking alcohol is not done indiscriminately, but is done within the ritual structure of a 'rite of passage' (Turner, 1967), where the use of alcohol is the key symbol for 'free flow' in the transition from childhood to the individual life project of creating one's social identity (Beccaria and Sande,

2003; Rolando, Beccaria, et al., 2012). As Douglas (in Wilson, 2005: 13) argues, 'drinking acts to mark the boundaries of personal and group identities, making it a practice of inclusion and exclusion'. Similarly, Wilson claims 'drinking activities are active elements in individual and group identifications, are the sites where drinking takes place, the locals of regular and celebrated drinking, are places where meanings are made, shared, disputed and reproduced, where identities take shape, flourish, change' (2005: 10).

Dwight Heath has spent several decades studying how different cultures use alcohol, and he maintains that there are predictable rules that operate in every culture that uses alcohol:

1. In most societies, drinking is a social act, embedded in a context of values, attitudes, and other norms.
2. These values, norms and attitudes influence the effects of drinking, regardless of how important biochemical, physiological and pharmokinetic factors may also be to the experience of drinking.
3. The drinking of alcoholic beverages tends to be hedged with rules. Often such rules are the focus of exceptionally strong emotions and sanctions.
4. The value of alcohol for promoting relaxation and sociability is emphasized in many populations and most populations treat alcohol intake as an act or celebration or something appropriate for celebrations.
5. The association of drinking with any kind of specifically associated problems is rare among cultures throughout both history and the contemporary world.
6. When alcohol-related problems do occur, they are clearly linked with modalities of drinking, and usually also with values, attitudes and norms about drinking. What is normal for consumption defines the abnormal that is considered a problem. Societies that consider drunkenness shameful or disgusting usually have less incidence of intoxication.
7. In cultures where drinking is considered heroic, masculine or desirable it tends to be embraced. These positive evaluations may provide little defence against the risks and dangers of excessive drinking.
8. Societies in which alcohol is disallowed to the young, and in which alcohol is considered to enhance the self by conferring sex appeal or power, tend to have youth who drink too much, too fast, for inappropriate or unrealistic reasons (Heath, 2000: 196–8).

Figure 1.2   The cultural patterning of alcohol use

As I develop in what follows, Heath's framework can be usefully deployed for understanding and interpreting sport-related drinking. As others have explored elsewhere (Palmer and Thompson, 2007; Clayton, 2012; 2008; Lake, 2012; McDonald and Sylvester, 2013), and indeed it is a point to which I return, drinking is central to a range of sports initiations and forms of socialisation and transition. Drinking is a membership norm of many amateur and professional sports, and it is often social convention to drink alcohol after practices, games and at other club or league related events (Collins and Vamplew, 2002: 101), yet curiously, this has hovered on the margins of interest from social anthropology, with ethnographic studies of sport-related drinking tending to focus instead on the 'carnivalesque' nature of major sporting events in which drinking is seen as an adjunct to the event more broadly rather than the central focus of the study being on drinking as an everyday social practice (Giulianotti, 1995; Millward, 2009). In other cases, such as Donnelly's (2013) account of drinking with the derby girls, drinking was a persistent backdrop to her ethnographic work with a group of roller derby players rather than the explicit focus of her wider analysis of roller derby as a particular social formation in late modernity.

Indeed, while anthropologists, sociologists and geographers, among others, have been acutely alert to the sociality and commensality of shared drinking in other empirical contexts, including office Christmas parties, Hen and Stag nights, backpacker tours, shore leave, university and college 'Fresher' or Orientation weeks, and school breaks, as well as the more traditional anthropological studies of ritualised drinking associated with various rites of passage, the social meanings that are shared and carried through drinking as it occurs in *sporting* contexts has been largely overlooked in these rich and fine-grained ethnographic analysis of drinking. As I elaborate in the following pages, alcohol serves as a symbolic vehicle for identifying and constructing cultural values in sport, for shaping social interactions and relationships in sport and for defining behavioural norms and expectations in sport.

This oversight, I'd suggest, is reflective of a broader trend in research that tends to distinguish studies of alcohol and other drugs from studies of drugs in sport, the latter having a focus on illicit and performance enhancing drugs, rather than the cultural dimensions of 'everyday' drug and alcohol use that I am concerned with here. This fairly arbitrary separation has meant that research into alcohol and other drugs, and research into drugs in sport have tended to operate as largely distinct fields, with little crossover of researchers, theoretical positions, methodological approaches or epistemological standpoints. This seems to be something of a missed opportunity, as both fields of research share similar interests and concerns. Both wrestle with definitions of drug and alcohol use and abuse, both must engage with the ethics of doing drug and alcohol research and the politics of drug policies, the stigmatisation and marginalisation of people for whom drug or alcohol use becomes problematic, the development and implementation of prevention and treatment strategies and the operation of harm reduction policies. Studies of alcohol and other drugs and studies of drugs in sport, in other words, can usefully learn from each other, and it is hoped that this book can contribute to a dialogue between the two fields of research.

From Drinking to Drunkenness

The sociality of sport-related drinking, like drinking elsewhere, is dependent on culture and context. Sports-associated drinking, like other forms of drinking, does not, take place just anywhere, and the book adopts the position that sport-related drinking is essentially a social act that is subject to a variety of rules and norms regarding who may drink what, when, where, why, how, with whom, and so on. The chapters in this first section of the book are thus primarily concerned to examine the cultural definitions and limitations that are placed on drinking in various sports and sporting contexts, as well as offering a way out of some of the existing theoretical limitations that constrain analyses.

While social anthropology and related disciplines have long had an interest in the social aspects of drinking, there has been a more recent shift from looking at the sociality of drinking to the social aspects of getting 'legless and pissy-arse falling down drunk' (Young, 1995), with studies of *drunkenness* becoming a key way we through which we can think about notions of becoming, belonging and other dimensions of sociality. As Cameron, et al. (2000) note in their study of intoxication across Europe, there has been a move away from questions of 'how much' to questions of 'what happened'; that is, what it felt like and what it meant to be very drunk in particular social situations.

There is a useful intellectual genealogy here. MacAndrew and Edgerton's (1969) *Drunken Comportment* provides an early ethnographic and historical account of drunken behaviour in different societies around the world that supports the argument that 'drunken comportment is culturally constructed or determined rather than pharmacologically determined' (Room, 1984). More recently, Measham's (2006) work in the United Kingdom describes cultural changes in the urban leisure scene where drinking to excess appears to be the whole purpose of, rather than ancillary to, a night out for young people, findings similarly reported by Lindsay (2009) in her study of drinking among youth in inner city Melbourne, Australia. These debates about the changing nature of leisure, the centrality of getting 'rat-arsed' or 'shit-faced', to use the Australian vernacular, and the problem of pleasure are revisited in the following chapter, which examines notions of calculated hedonism, determined drunkenness and hegemonic drinking as alternative theoretical frameworks for understanding 'drunken comportment' as it occurs in particular sporting contexts.

While studies of drunkenness can be and are immensely revealing of aspects of social life, they are not without their problems. As Beccaria and Sande note 'alcohol for the purposes of intoxication and drunkenness can be seen as a social practice presenting theoretical and methodological challenges for social sciences' (2003: 100). The ethics of doing research with people who are inebriated, how to write about this behaviour without being seen to valorise it or alternatively, without responding to it as a moral panic deserving of a swift (and usually uncritical) policy response, and whether we are sufficiently equipped theoretically to understand and explain drunkenness in sport or elsewhere, are all considered in the following chapters.

While drinking, and drinking to excess, carries considerable normative currency in sport, it would be disingenuous to suggest that this is always the case. As I explore in Chapter 4, non-drinkers are becoming more and more conspicuous in high-level sport, with religious beliefs and notions of care of the self and physical austerity by athletes being key factors here. Nonetheless 'binge' or 'extreme' drinking as it is variously (and not unproblematically) known is the conceptual architecture on which popular understandings and indeed many first-hand experiences of sport-related drinking are typically hung, and it is important to subject experiences of drunkenness to sustained critical, *theoretical* scrutiny rather than to rely on anecdote alone.

Extreme Drinking

In recent years, media and policy attention has highlighted 'binge' drinking as a social problem [where] the 'focus of concern has been on young people's drinking and on the behaviours and harms associated with it in relation to public health, public safety and public order' (Esenbach-Stangl and Thom, 2009: 1). Variously defined as 'heroic drinking', 'extreme drinking' (Glassman, Todd, et al., 2010, and 'coma drinking' in German speaking countries, the term 'binge drinking' is commonly used to describe drinking where the threshold exceeds five or more drinks for men and four or more for women per occasion (NHMRC, 2001). While 'binge' or 'extreme' drinking as it occurs in sporting contexts is revisited in the following chapter, and again in Chapters 6 and 8 in terms of both the practice then the policy responses, it is important to note here that such terminology is far from straightforward. One UK Home Office publication, for example, described a 'binge drinker' as someone who reported "feeling very drunk once a month"' (Richardson and Budd, 2003) while an alternative definition describes it as an individual drinking over a day or more until unconscious (Newburn and Shiner, 2001).

Such definitions are further problematised by the fact that the alcohol content of drinks varies, particularly across international definitions of what constitutes a standard drink, the length of time in a drinking occasion or a sitting is not defined, and the clinical definition of a binge differs from that used in the social sciences (where it might be described as a bender), which differs again from the way in which the term is used colloquially, where getting 'pissed', 'ratted', 'rat-arsed', 'legless', 'shit-faced', 'wasted' or 'wrecked' are among the more popular expressions used to describe single occasion drinking (Cameron, 2000) deemed to be risky or problematic.

This is an important point, for it is widely assumed and theorised that heavy, problematic, drinking is an integral part of sporting identities, cultures and practices (O'Brien, Ali, et al. 2007). As is addressed in Chapter 4, however, this is not always the case. The demographic profile of many sports has changed through migration, ethnic diversity, and religion and faith, which have led to increasing numbers of sportsmen (and women), as well as sports fans, abstaining from alcohol consumption. While a discussion of non-drinking may seem odd in a book on drinking, it is important to include a discussion of non-drinkers; that is, sportsmen and women, as well as sports fans who consciously choose not to drink for whatever reason, for it allows an exploration of contradictory identities in sports cultures and relationships that, to date, have eluded discussion and debate. As I explore in Chapter 4, asking questions of what people *don't* do (i.e. electing not to drink) can be just as revealing as interrogating what people actually do, and the negative case of non-drinkers in an environment where strong normative codes of drinking prevail allows an exploration of questions of legitimacy, authenticity, belonging, health and bodycare, among other things, in ways that extend the theoretical and empirical contributions to studies of sport and alcohol.

While there is some equivocation as to the definition of 'binge' drinking, extreme drinking in sport, and more broadly, does seem to be something of a Western problem. We see very little research coming out of the Global South or from BRIC countries (the acronym for Brazil, Russia, India and China) in relation to problem drinking and sport. This may be a hangover (no pun intended) of what Hunt and Barker (2001) and Room (1984) have previously referred to as a 'problem deflation', whereby anthropologists have 'systematically underestimated the extent of alcohol problems in Third World societies' (Hunt and Barker, 2001: 167), or in which 'anthropologists tend to minimize the seriousness of drinking problems in the tribal and village cultures under discussion' (Room, 1984: 170). Although referring to a fairly traditional version of anthropological inquiry that has more recently been complemented by studies of fully globalised, developed, Western cultural milieux, the concerns raised do highlight something of a gap in research on drinking, and drinking problems, sport-related or otherwise, as it occurs in non-Western settings.

Equally, this, in part, is reflective of a lack of national-level drug and alcohol data collected from BRIC countries or those in the Global South where data is more often collected through partial and/or local-level surveys being undertaken by non-government organisations. As such, it is difficult to capture a complete picture of the prevalence of drug and alcohol use and misuse in these countries or, indeed, the ways in which sport-related drinking features in country profiles of alcohol consumption.

Given this caveat about limited data, I examine briefly examines some of the harm *reduction* (as distinct from harm minimisation) strategies that have been implemented in Japan, Thailand and Brazil. In their work on alcohol harm reduction in Brazil, Gorgulho and Da Ros (2006) caution about falling into the trap of stereotypical assumptions as to who a 'problem drinker' is. While they note that such assumptions are frequently universal; that is, a 'problem drinker' is assumed to be unemployed and/or of low socio-economic status and with lower levels of educational attainment, Gorgulho and Da Ros (2006) warn that 'one should take care with such an assumption, since levels of alcohol consumption are also very high among Brazil's middle class and well-educated young people' (2006: 35).

While these are not specific to sport-related drinking, they do raise questions and concerns for the global sports landscape, and the broader cultural context which sees a number of sporting mega-events being hosted by cities and BRIC countries and the Global South, such as the 2014 Winter Olympics in Sochi, the 2016 Summer Olympics in Rio de Janeiro, or the 2022 World Cup in Qatar. In light of this, the intersections between sport, alcohol and 'the global ecumene' (Hannerz, 1989) are critical concerns. The implications of hosting major events in traditionally 'dry' regions such as the Gulf States are addressed further in Chapter 4 where the issue of non-drinkers and sport is explored, and the cross-cultural aspects of health promotion and prevention initiatives are considered more fully in Chapter 8.

The implications of this broader policy focus on extreme drinking and drunkenness are several-fold, and are these are elaborated further in the following chapters. Briefly though, notwithstanding (or perhaps because of) the health costs and consequences of binge drinking, it is regarded as problematic by a growing band of health and policy professionals because of the perceived normalisation of the behaviour. A number of scholars note that what was once pathologised as harmful or 'risky' drinking is now considered par for the course among young drinkers in particular, with drinking that fits the definition of 'binge drinking' being seen simply a part of a night out for many (Demant and Bruvik-Heinskou, 2011).

While this is a point dealt with more fully in the second half of the book, it is worth noting here that the banalisation or normalisation of extreme drinking in sport or more broadly has very real costs and consequences. There is no shortage of literature, research or media reporting describing the effects of acute alcohol-related harms in terms of accidents, injuries, hospitalisations, violence, assaults and, in some cases, fatalities. While the focus, for the most part, has been on data reflecting male drinking behaviours, this can be, in part, explained by a return to particular assumptions that cast men, sport and alcohol are something of a 'holy trinity' (Wenner and Jackso, 2009). As Peralta and Jauk ask, somewhat rhetorically, 'perhaps it is because men are at greater risk for alcohol-related problems (both perpetrating and experiencing) that research on alcohol has taken men and masculinity for granted – as "natural" and therefore normal' (2011: 890). Increasingly, however, public health and policy concern with binge drinking involved women, where females drinking in public, in particular, provokes a wider social anxiety. This debate, and its application to sport-related drinking, is explored further in Chapter 3.

The normalisation of extreme drinking in sport and more broadly also alerts us to a shift in policy focus and discourse from drinking that is damaging or 'risky' to drinking that is fun, pleasurable and 'normal'. This shift is by no means unique to alcohol consumption. Since the end of the 1980s, risky behaviours, among young people in particular, have become a major issue for public health. As Pike notes in relation to the development of a major sexual health strategy in the United Kingdom, 'once a situation is defined as risky, it is then also political, since governments and individuals are required to attend to it' (2007: 311).

Along with smoking, using recreational drugs or practicing unsafe sex, drinking continues to command considerable attention as one of the behaviours practiced by young people that are perceived to put their health at risk. Several studies have looked at drinking games, where large amounts of – often high alcohol content – drinks are consumed rapidly. Jayne, et al. (2010), for example, have examined the phenomenon among groups of backpackers, and certainly, there are a number of initiations into sporting clubs that involve drinking games of one sort or another (Palmer and Thompson, 2007; Palmer, 2009; Clayton, 2012; Lake, 2012; McDonald and Sylvester, 2013).

Beccaria and Sande (2003: 101) argue – fairly dramatically – that drinking games inside peer groups are a form of practice that involve playing with the limits between intoxication and death; yet among those who take part in the activity, this is rarely at the front of their minds, where the objective risk of taking part in an activity has been stripped from the subjective experience of those who engage in it. Dobson, et al. (2006), for example, followed a group of Norwegian youth who were in their in the final year of high school who pursued a number of activities that were considered 'normless and regarded as a necessary part of being a so-called *russ* [a final year high school student]' (Dobson et al, 2006: 50). While many of the *russ* activities were clearly dangerous (e.g. sleeping on a roadway traffic island), the behaviours of participants were only considered to be courting risk by those who were outside of the activities. For those taking part, however, the activities were necessary rites of passage marking the end of high school and the transition into the adult world. This conflicting discourse is a point to which I'll return in subsequent chapters, for it presents a major challenge for policy and practice across a number of policy sectors from crime and social order to health and wellbeing. Understanding and balancing the tensions between the 'fun' of collective drinking – in sport or elsewhere – with the real (and potential) costs and consequence is a challenge to policy-makers (Jayne, Holloway and Valentine, 2006: 463), and the implications of this for research, policy and practice are points to which the book will variously return.

Some Early Notes on Policy and Practice

The socially constructed nature of policy problems, solutions and interventions is a theme that runs through much of my research, and I've examined elsewhere the role of human intervention in policy formulation and failures in a range of sporting contexts (Palmer, 2013c). While many of the implications and interventions of public policy (broadly defined) for sport-related drinking are addressed in the second half of this book, some preliminary observations are needed here for they provide an important background to some of the debates about policy emphases and effectiveness that continue to gain traction in modern, democratic societies.

To set up the argument, my focus is less on the exceptional or 'extreme' actions and behaviours that characterise crisis-driven policy making as it relates to alcohol consumption, and more on the everyday nature of sport-related drinking. By that, I mean that alcohol consumption is often cast as an extreme or an exceptional problem, and most policy has developed in response to various health and social crises. As Eisnebach-Stangl and Thom note public attention 'ties and bundles scientific attention, and imprints the landscape of social research by defining the most acute problems, by influencing the questions asked and the financial means given to scientists to explore these questions' (2009: 20).

As I suggested earlier however, sport-related drinking is not always excessive or exceptional, much of it is in fact quite mundane, and it is the ways in which it is experienced, practiced, understood and articulated that are the central concerns of the book. That is, I am interested to chart the 'normal and everyday use of these substances, with their attendant rituals, customs and paraphernalia within social and cultural contexts' (Hunt and Barker, 2001: 171).

Nonetheless, much of the sport/alcohol policy debate is embedded in a wider social anxiety about extreme drinking, and with the drinking done by women and young people more specifically. In particular, much policy attention is given over to mitigating the harms and consequences of alcohol consumption in the night-time economy where various policies and strategies have been put in place to militate against 'binge' drinking. In Australia and the United Kingdom, for example, pubs and clubs now operate with extended licensing hours to offset the pressure to 'drink up' at closing time, and certainly, much of sport-related drinking can be thought of as part of the night-time economy or as 'part-time deviance' (Aldridge, et al., 2011).

As a consequence, a considerable focus of alcohol-related policy focuses on public safety and reducing violence, yet, to return to a theme from earlier, reducing violence or removing the risk is a delicate balancing act between maintaining order and control and not stifling the very conditions that attract so many people (Hobbs, et al., 2003). In his work on youth drinking, Tutenges (2009), for example, notes that in one Bulgarian nightclub, there were insufficient safety measures in place – patrons could dance on furniture, shattered glass lay on the floor, and the venue was overcrowded, among other things – yet the heavy drinking youth in attendance were largely unaware of these inadequate safety measures or the potential consequences.

While harm reduction 'up to a point' seems to be the conventional wisdom in thinking about constructing alcohol policy, such strategies and the focus on the night-time economy and reducing the impacts of drinking in licensed venues or in public spaces in particular (Jayne, Holloway and Valentine, 2006), may be of little value when the drinking can start at 10am in the morning or earlier, and where domestic drinking and pre-loading are increasingly part of the drinking practices associated with attending and viewing sports matches (Holloway, Jayne and Valentine, 2008). Indeed, sport-related drinking is increasingly being done during the day and in private homes (friends gathering to watch a major game on a Saturday afternoon, for example) which lie beyond the policy gaze. While these are points to which I will return, parallels can be drawn with the 'home alone' parties in Norway, where groups of friends contribute to the small scale production of home distilled spirits (*hjemmebrent*) that are then drunk to celebrate major events such as birthdays, and more mundane occasions such as finishing a domestic task (Beccaria and Sande, 2003). Indeed, much of sport and the drinking that goes with it, takes place during the day in quite ordinary and mundane ways.

Similarly, while much research on drinking has focussed on drinking in cities as part of a project of modernity, as integral to the construction of identity in club cultures (Thornton, 2005; Hutton, 2004) or as part of youth cultures (McRobbie, 1994; Measham, Aldridge, et al. 2001), drinking in rural and regional communities is a major in concern in countries like Canada and New Zealand and Chapter 6 reviews some of the initiatives that are in place in relation to sport-related drinking to counter some of the harms and damages of drinking outside of urban centres.

Alongside this, much of the policy agenda of alcohol consumption is crucially linked to economic savings and to health benefits. The sale and distribution of alcohol, for example, is regulated, predominantly by means of taxation or through a State-owned liquor monopolies and licensing systems that limit the sale and distribution of alcohol to liquor stores (Beccaria and Sande, 2003; Higuchi, Matsushita and Osaki, 2006), or through initiatives that restrict off-premise retail sales, impose minimum legal drinking ages, enforce penalties for drink driving or that drive up the price through taxation. While measures such as the use of price, taxation, and availability are recognised as evidence based approaches to reducing alcohol-related harm, these provide the policy background to rather than the focus of the book. That said, although the book is not intended as a policy book, it cannot sidestep the importance of understanding the behaviour and cultural practices that inform policy. While policy emphases may shift, central themes persist and these underscore much of the analysis of sport-related drinking elaborated in the following pages.

The fundamental question of how advanced consumer societies balance individual freedom of choice with the need to manage and prevent alcohol and other drug problems is not easily resolved, for effective policies such as reducing the availability of alcohol or increasing the cost of high strength alcohol impact on consumer choice, on market freedom and on lifestyle issues that are considered to be private matters. Thus, policy solutions often emphasise the moral management of the self, but this may lead to the moral management of 'the other'. While this argument is typically espoused in relation to young people and other populations deemed to be 'at-risk', drinkers in sport are commonly perceived as problem 'others', with sport-related drinking associated with a raft of social and health problems and celebrity infamy which makes it a policy problem in and of itself.

A Note on Theories and Methods

It is not intended that this book be read as a research monograph, rather a commentary on the key themes and gaps in research on sport-related drinking. Although grounded in some of my empirical research on Australian Rules football, the book also draws on primary research (interviews and participant-observation) and secondary analyses of biographical and autobiographical material from sportsmen and women involved with other codes of football (i.e. rugby, soccer), or with cricket, Ultimate Frisbee, roller derby and hockey, snooker and golf, along with sporting mega-events such as the Olympic Games or football's World Cup. Equally, readings of the 'grey' literature and key policy documents are used to advance the central arguments of the book. Thus, the material assembled is a deliberately diverse and eclectic selection that reflects my previous, current or emerging research interests in relation to sport and drinking practices. Given this, the chapters, where relevant, include a brief methodological statement and overview of how the data that informs the chapter was collected and analysed.

Although the book is diverse and interdisciplinary in terms of the empirical studies and it draws on my critical interpretivist background as a social anthropologist, and the empirical data that is reported is thus largely qualitative and socio-cultural in nature. As is the case with much of my other work, my approach here is characterised by 'a healthy disrespect for disciplinary boundaries, an adventurous cross-cultural curiosity and a commitment to critical social scientific scholarship not beholden to patrons, agencies or sponsors' (Sugden and Tomlinson, 2011: xiii).

While qualitative and ethnographic approaches to studies of drug, alcohol and sporting cultures are no longer original and their contribution to the field are well recognised (Agar, 1973; Moore and Maher, 2002; Neale, Allen and Coombes, 2005; Weed, 2006), ethnographic approaches to *drinking in the context of sport* are curiously under-researched. Where they have been adopted, analyses have tended to reproduce the theoretical orthodoxies and taken-for-granted positions that this book seeks to move beyond (Armstrong and Hognestad, 2006; Ayers and Treadwell, 2012). In noting this gap, I am not suggesting so much that scholars are failing to investigate particular issues, rather that there are relatively few qualitative researcher or ethnographers working on issues of sport and alcohol as a myriad cultural phenomenon, and it is this gap in the research that this book is intended to redress.

In keeping with the spirit of qualitative research, much of the book is concerned with describing the 'social meanings that participants attach to their [alcohol use and misuse], and the social processes by which such meanings are created, reinforced and reproduced' (Neale, et al., 2005: 1584). I am particularly concerned in unravelling how and why sport-related drinking practices can be understood in different contexts and among different social groups (Rhodes, 1995; Nichter, et al., 2004). The value of qualitative approaches is particularly notable when considering *non-drinkers* and sport. For the most part, studies have been quantitative, comparative or cross-sectional, and have tended to examine rates of non-drinking in relation to drinking among particular population cohorts such as college students and student athletes. While useful for identifying patterns and prevalence in a broader adult population, missing from such studies are the non-drinkers' accounts of the social context or the 'definitions of the situation' (Thomas, 1937 in Herman-Kinney and Kinney, 2012: 4) in which non-drinking occurs. An analysis of the 'definitions of the situation' among non-drinkers forms the backdrop to Chapter 4.

It is worth noting as well that the book engages with many of the methodological and epistemological debates on the 'movement to technique' in qualitative research in drug and alcohol research. By this, I mean researchers have been critical of the increasing separation of qualitative methods from their theoretical framework in drug research (Bourgois, 1999; 2002; Moore, 2002; Moore and Maher, 2002). That is, there is a focus on the nuts and bolts – the pragmatic realities – of doing qualitative research among drug and alcohol users, rather than due attention to theoretical frameworks that can inform the practice of qualitative social research, and the analyses that are then extrapolated from this. As I return to in the following chapter and elsewhere, theory is needed to critically interrogate the taken-for-granted orthodoxies that have dominated perceptions of sport-related drinking in the public realm; most notably, that it is a bastion of hegemonic masculinity.

My focus on theoretically informed empirical qualitative research does, however, alert us to a body of scholarship that this book does not engage with extensively. The relationship between sport and alcohol in terms of marketing and promotional culture is a significant one; a substantial body of research explores the ways in which many of the commercials associated with alcohol sponsorship in sport reproduce particular constructions of identity, for example, and advertising, in particular, is increasingly regarded as a strategic medium for analysis because of its pivotal role in linking production with consumption in the circuit of culture (du Gay et al., 1997; Jackson, Andrews and Scherer, 2005; Scherer and Jackson, 2008; Wenner and Jackson, 2009). In analysing this circuit of culture, however, there is something of a methodological predilection for text-based analyses of images and representations, with more empirical, primary research such as interviews, surveys, focus groups or observation being relatively side lined, and an ethnographic treatment of the circuit of sport-related promotional culture warrants a book in itself. Empirical research with producers and consumers of alcohol advertising in sport would usefully complement these largely semiotic readings of the text, although these are beyond the scope of this current book, and I acknowledge the gap.

Equally, while this book is offered as something of a riposte to the theoretical emphases of hegemonic masculinity that dominate analyses of sport-related drinking, I have not replaced this with a singular theoretical framework as an alternative. Instead, I adopt something of a *bricoleur* approach; applying those theories that are most adept to explain the context, circumstances and behaviours under study. That is, the book takes its theoretical lead from the empirical case studies it presents.

Given the complexity of the sport-alcohol nexus and the breadth of material it encompasses, I recognise a number of ways in which we might rethink drinking and sport as being a diffuse cultural phenomenon that mediates or acts as a conduit for all kinds of social relationships. On this, I follow Wheaton who argues that

> such an approach that uses theory as a tool box, "heurist device" (e.g. Pearson, 1981), or framework for understanding cultural phenomenon is an approach

that some theorists find problematic. However, being open to a diversity of theoretical interpretations, as well as methodological approaches, enables the researcher to provide a more vivid picture of the complex and shifting cultural phenomenon under study (2013: 8).

As the book is an attempt to widen the empirical, theoretical and conceptual base upon which studies of sport-related drinking have typically been located, it reflects the theoretical eclecticism of the field in elaborating the key argument of each subsequent chapter.

Conclusion

This chapter has been concerned to sketch out some of the key concepts and debates in the sport-alcohol nexus, particularly how they inform the analytical framework of this book, namely the three-way consideration of the popular imaginings of sport-related drinking, under-represented relationships between sport and alcohol and the relationships between sport, alcohol, treatment and prevention. This provides the overarching dynamic within which to consider the material developed in the rest of the book. That said, this framework is best thought of as just that – a framework. A more nuanced elaboration of the key concepts and debates introduced here is needed to consider the complex, contested and contradictory nature of drinking – and drinkers in sport. One of the central themes put forward is that sport-related drinking is essentially a social act, albeit done in different ways, with different meanings, implications and consequences depending on the drinker and the context in which drinking occurs. With that in mind, the following chapter begins to move the debate beyond 'hegemonic masculinity', and explores the notion of drinking as 'contested leisure' as a way of recasting and extending the theoretical debate on the nature of sport-related drinking and people's experiences, understandings and articulations of this relationship.

Chapter 2

Beyond Hegemonic Masculinity: Social Theory and Sport-related Drinking

> This chapter:
> - examines the application of key theoretical frameworks to studies of sport-related drinking;
> - reviews the literature on sport, alcohol and hegemonic masculinity;
> - posits the notion of hegemonic *drinking* as a new way of rethinking drinking and sport.

Introduction

One of the arguments developed in this book is that sociological accounts of sport-related drinking have tended to be done within a fairly limited theoretical framework, in doing so, maintaining a series of established orthodoxies that orient the analysis of drinking in sport in particular ways. As I suggested in the previous chapter, sport-related drinking, particularly heavy drinking, is more often than not conceptualised as a 'bastion of masculinity' where drinking practices are theorised through the lens of 'hegemonic masculinity', drawing on the influential work of the Australian sociologist Raewyn Connell. While Connell's contributions to the field are assuredly significant – there are few other terms or concepts in the social sciences, I'd suggest, that have attracted such widespread and sustained interest – the assumptions and orientations inherent in such framings nonetheless obscure or miss entirely other theoretical frameworks through which sport-related drinking might be explained, interpreted or analysed. As I argue in this chapter, analyses of the sport-alcohol nexus can be strengthened by the application of social theory, drawn from the social sciences more broadly.

I have suggested elsewhere (Palmer, 2013a) that social scientists with an interest in drinking beyond sport have seen the possibilities of a range of theoretical frameworks for explaining the cultural practices, the social interactions and, indeed, the consequences, of consuming alcohol. Drawing on these may lead to a more nuanced understanding of *sport*-related drinking, and it is these that I tease out in the following pages.

Theorising drinking in the context of sport is important for a number of reasons. Relative to sociological or anthropological studies of food, which have attracted the attention of major social theorists (such as Pierre Bourdieu or Mary Douglas), theorising *drinking*, particularly sport-related drinking, suffers from something of an ambivalence about the legitimacy of focussing on alcohol as a subject of study (Singer, 1986: 114), particularly when it is so solidly framed as a social problem or a policy problem. As I noted in the preface, one of my concerns is to move beyond the deficit model of conceptualising sport-related drinking as a 'problem', but we require a more developed set of theoretical possibilities to help explain both the everyday as well as the exceptional or problematic aspects of sport-related drinking.

Returning to a concern with the 'movement to technique' in qualitative research in drug and alcohol research, I would suggest that where particular research methods have been deployed to explain aspects of sport-related drinking, theory has been largely absent from the analysis. Quantitative work such as surveys (i.e. the technique) tends to describe prevalence among or comparisons of alcohol consumption between particular cohorts (sports science students make popular subjects), and theory of any kind is almost entirely absent. Where qualitative methods have been employed (and I include some of my own work here), this has been done in terms of the kinds of theoretically limited ways this book is keen to move beyond. Thus, a key challenge is how to undertake empirically rich, theoretically sophisticated research in ways that can truly reflect the complexity and diversity of sport-related drinking and drinkers.

From this starting point, my concern in this chapter is to sketch out some alternative conceptual frameworks for explaining (and critiquing) sport-related drinking in order to identify some of the research avenues these may then open up for policy, practice and debate. There are, of course, multiple versions of sociological theory that could contribute to studies of sport-related drinking and, in this chapter I examine just four key theoretical perspectives from sociology that have much currency in studies of drug and alcohol use more broadly in order to suggest their application to studies of sport-related drinking. These are:

1. the notions of determined drunkenness and calculated hedonism;
2. Pierre Bourdieu's application of symbolic capital within the framework of distinction;
3. the 'normalisation' theory popular in socio-criminological studies of drug use, particularly among young people, and;
4. Michel Foucault's work on disciplinary power.

I've chosen these perspectives, not because they are representative in any way, rather because they represent the 'ongoing need to reassess and reinvigorate the theoretical frameworks that drive drug research, policy and practice' (Moore and Rhodes, 2006: 324).

With this as background, this chapter unfolds in the following way. It begins by reviewing the literature on sport, alcohol and hegemonic masculinity as the theoretical starting point for most analyses of sport-related drinking. It then moves on to a consideration of the four alternative theoretical perspectives that could usefully be applied to studies of sport-related drinking, before positing the notion of hegemonic *drinking*, rather than masculinity, as a new way of rethinking drinking and sport.

Sport, Alcohol and Hegemonic Masculinity

Sport and drinking have long been regarded as among the more routine, yet problematic, sites where notions of masculinity are played out. While there is no shortage of scholarly interest in either masculinity and sport or masculinity and alcohol, my concern in this chapter is to extend rather than revisit that literature. That said, a brief review of some of the research on drinking alcohol and masculinity more broadly is perhaps needed, for it foregrounds (and replicates) some of the theoretical positions adopted when considering sport-related drinking more specifically.

The relationship between 'socially condoned practices of drinking alcohol and the social construction and performance of masculine identities in the 20th century is well noted' (Thurnell-Read, 2012: 3). The consumption of alcohol and the successful enactment of drinking (and drunkenness) is widely regarded in Western, neoliberal and democratic societies as being among the quintessential or archetypical practices through which particular forms of masculine identity can be explored, enacted and embodied (Gough and Edwards, 1998; De Visser and McDonnell, 2012; Campbell, 2000; Thurnell-Read, 2011a; 2011b; 2012; Dempster, 2011). As Hunt, et al. succinctly put it, 'to drink is to be masculine and to be drunk is to be even more masculine' (Hunt, et al., 2005: 227).

There are a number of empirical and geographical contexts in which the relationship between the embodiment or physical expression of drinking and masculinity has been explored. Thurnell-Read, in his discussion of a Stag Tour in Krakow, notes that alcohol is closely related to masculine embodiment in that 'drinking practices, and the spaces in which they take place, offer many men a means to performatively sustain their masculine identity' (2011a: 979). Similarly, Campbell's work on drinking among male pub goers in rural New Zealand elaborates what he describes as 'conversational cockfighting' (2000: 565). Among the drinkers in Campbell's ethnographic study, verbal sparring and the trading of light hearted insults demonstrate a kind of masculine mastery in which drinking serves as a source of legitimising and validation for masculine identity, as well as a space in which to perform particular notions of a particular kind of masculinity (Campbell, 2000: 566). As Peralta and Jauk ask, somewhat rhetorically, 'perhaps it is because men are at greater risk for alcohol-related problems (both perpetrating and experiencing) that research on alcohol has taken men and masculinity for granted – as "natural" and therefore normal' (2011: 890).

As noted already, many of these studies on the masculine nature of drinking (and sport) owe their intellectual legacy to the Australian sociologist Raewyn Connell. Inspired, in turn, by the work of Antonio Gramsci, Connell argues that within any given social context a particular hierarchy to gender relations exists, where the 'gender order' is structured by a hegemonic form of masculinity (Pringle, 2011). Associated with whiteness, heterosexuality, authority, toughness and competitiveness, hegemonic masculinity, as a 'state or condition of ideology, frames understandings of how particular ways of performing maleness seem natural and normal, yet at the same time act to sustain problematic relations of dominance within and between males and females' (Pringle, 2011: 111).

Such observations resonate with studies of sport-related drinking cultures. Curry's (1998; 2000) descriptive work on team dynamics within American college athletic teams, for example, identifies a strong, normative culture of heavy drinking among male athletes, as does Black, Lawson and Fleishman's (1999) research on rugby league in Australia. The role of alcohol in football-related disorder has also been noted (Williams, et al., 1989; King, 1997) and parallels can be drawn with other boisterous spectator groups such as the 'Barmy Army' (Parry and Malcolm, 2004).[1]

Equally, my own work on 'the Grog Squad' (Palmer and Thompson, 2007; Palmer, 2009) or Clayton and Harris' (2008) discussion of 'our friend Jack' provides further empirical evidence of the masculine nature of drinking and sport. Key to Clayton and Harris work is an analysis of the ritual practices of initiation among a male university rugby team in the south of England, while my work explored the drinking-based behaviours, practices and interactions of an exclusively male Australian Rules football supporter group where 'belonging, identity and social status revolved around spectacularly high levels of alcohol consumption' (Palmer and Thompson, 2007: 188). A key theme in each of these accounts is that drinking is attributed to 'being a man', where being able to drink, and to 'drink well' in terms of the quantity and the pace of alcohol consumption, along with the management of physical symptoms and bodily control, enables the enactment of socially ascribed ideals of masculinity (Peralta, 2007; Leyshon, 2005).

While hegemonic masculinity continues to serve as the dominant paradigm for understanding and theorising men's attitudes, behaviours and practices in sport (and when drinking), scholars are increasingly recognising that *masculinities* (plural) are a contested concept (Flood, 2002; 2008; McKay, Messner and Sabo, 2000; Pringle, 2005). Anderson (2005; 2009), for example, distinguishes hegemonic masculinity from *orthodox* masculinity, arguing that 'scholars frequently confuse Connell's notion of hegemonic masculinity as a social process with the archetype described as maintaining social dominance' (Adams, Anderson and McCormack, 2010: 280), and it is the presentation of the archetype that is esteemed in sporting cultures as orthodox masculinity.

Similarly, Seidler (2006) and Thorpe (2010) suggest that hegemonic masculinity is a blunt theoretical tool that has not kept pace with the gender order

---

1   The 'Barmy Army' is the name given to the group of English cricket fans who follow the Test series around the globe. The name was given to the group by the Australian media during the 1994–1995 Test series in Australia, for the group's willingness to travel to Australia in the near certain knowledge that the English team would lose.

and the fluidity of gender relations and identities in sport and elsewhere. Seidler, in particular, states that the theory is simply out-dated:

> We need to be aware of how gender relations have transformed within patriarchal cultures … . This does not imply that patriarchal relations have disappeared or that violence against women or gays has lessened, but such relations do not carry the same legitimacy for young people who have grown up within very different gender and sexual orders (2006: 3).

While Seidler is critical of the a-historical use of hegemonic masculinity, others (Connell herself included) have attempted to rework the concept so as to acknowledge hegemonic masculinit*ies*, and the intersectoral relationships between gender and race, class and ethnicity (Connell and Messerschmidt, 2005; Beasley, 2008; Schippers, 2007).

Such recognition of the complexity of masculinities, however, only serves to underscore the limitations with which the masculine nature of *sport-related drinking* has been considered. While a growing sensitivity to the complexity of men and their relationships vis-à-vis sport (or alcohol) is important, it does highlight a number of gaps, including the almost total absence of literature on women, sport and alcohol, on non-drinkers and 'light' or social drinkers and sport, as well as older men, gay men, non-Anglo men and other males who sit outside of normative assumptions of men in sport. Indeed, the construction of sport and drinking as a bastion of masculinity tends to flatten men, and masculinity, into something of a homogeneous category, whereas the plurality of men, and their relationships to sport and alcohol may, in fact, be far more nuanced.

Following on from this, Demetriou (2005) draws a distinction between 'internal' hegemonic masculinity and 'external' hegemonic masculinity, suggesting that hegemonic masculinity can be both the valuing of masculinity and the legitimising of male authority. It is this recognition of a relational dimension through the exercise of male authority over women and among different kinds of men that studies of sport-related drinking have not adequately addressed. Central to the argument developed in this chapter is that sport-related drinking is more than just the enactment and embodiment of normative gendered behaviours and we need to develop a more sophisticated theoretical framework through which to think about the complexity and contradictions of drinking and drinkers in sporting contexts. It is a consideration of some alternative theoretical positions that this chapter turns to now.

Determined Drunkenness, Calculated Hedonism and Extreme Drinking

In the last 20 years, researchers have sought to rethink drinking, particularly among youth and young adults in the context of late neoliberalism and the night-time economy (Brain, 2000; Griffin, Bengry-Howell, et al., 2009; Measham,

2004a; 2004b; Szmigin et al., 2008). As Brain notes, in this post-industrial consumer-oriented domain, individuals are able – and expected – to pursue pleasure and gratification through direct consumption. At the same time, however, neoliberal discourses that emphasise 'care of the self' (Foucault, 1988), and locate responsibilities for problems such as alcohol misuse with individuals rather than society have simultaneously become dominant, particularly in media accounts of 'the problem' (Measham and Brain, 2005; Griffin, Bengry-Howell, et al., 2009). As Brain notes, 'there is an evident tension' (2009: 12) insofar as discourses of consumerism encourage the pursuit of pleasure, while discourses of self-care emphasise moderation and restraint. Of concern for this chapter, heavy sessional or 'binge' drinkers, and young drinkers more particularly, are routinely subject to scrutiny from media, health authorities and governments for their excessive consumption of alcohol without seeming to recognise these tensions (Hayward and Hobbs, 2007; Szmigin, et al., 2008).

While this discursive disjuncture is a point to which I return in Chapter 8, it is important to note here that while a Foucauldian analysis (also addressed later in the chapter) seeks to situate the individual drinker within a 'regulated freedom' (Rose and Miller, 1992: 174) that emphasises the ways in which individual subjects (drinkers in this case) are located within notions of restraint and self-control (i.e. government of the self) and governmental constraints, such as alcohol taxes and levies (Dean, 1994; Foucault, 1988), a body of research seeks to situate drinkers not in terms of their interactions with governmental regulation and constraint, but in a broader context of pre-mediated pleasure and consumption or 'determined drunkenness' (Griffin, Bengry-Howell, et al., 2009) in which drinking to excess is tempered by calculated choices about where, when, how and what to drink.

Brain's research in the United Kingdom, for example, suggested that drinkers organised their drinking around other commitments such as school, work or family. In this way, Brain's research participants were what he termed 'calculated hedonists' (2000: 9), in that they sought 'sensuous indulgence of consuming but always in planned, carefully controlled ways' (2000: 9). Described by Featherstone (1994) as a form of liminal experience in which the individual strategically moves in and out of control, the idea of calculated de-control should not be equated with losing control, but with

> the capacity of the subject (in this case, the drinker) to modern subject to strategically "de-control" the emotions – to be open to an extended range of sensations and to enjoy shifting between the pleasures of attachment and of detached distance (Fenwick and Hayward, 2000: 46).

Similarly, Measham found that young drinkers (and drug users) planned and controlled their consumption 'within the boundaries of time (the weekend), space (club, bar, private party), company (supportive friends) and intensity' (2004a: 319). Jayne, et al.'s (2012) work with backpackers echoes this notion of a 'controlled loss of control' (Measham, 2002: 319). Drawing on empirical research conducted in Australia, Jayne, et al. (2012) argue that drinking and drunkenness are key components of backpacking holidays, shaping the rhythm of travel through the spatial and temporal imperatives of 'passing the time' and 'being able to do nothing' as well as heightening a sense of belonging with both fellow travellers and the 'locals' they encounter in bars, pubs, clubs and the like.

Notions of calculated hedonism and determined drunkenness have much resonance with sports-associated drinking. Sport is peppered with examples of a pre-mediated loss of control. End-of-season drinking trips, booze cruises, pub crawls, drinking safaris, 'skulling' competitions and 'boat races', alcohol-fuelled celebrations and commiserations and tours by football fans to 'previously unknown European cities which carried a "legend" dimension where hedonistic activities such as collective binge drinking' (Millward, 2009: 388) are all illustrative of the determined drunkenness that prevails in many sporting clubs. That is, they are displays of planned and pre-meditated excess that characterise calculated hedonism.[2]

Notions of calculated hedonism or determined drunkenness also resonate with Gordon, et al.'s (2012) depiction of 'fiesta drunkenness'. Defined as 'sporadic extreme drunkenness', fiesta drunkenness is closely tied to pleasure and celebration where getting 'out of it' is the deliberate and pre-mediated end game. In terms of sport-related drinking, McDonald and Sylvester's (2013) work on initiations into Japanese university sporting clubs describes the ways in which learning to drink, to drink to excess, and to drink in culturally prescribed ways, are all crucially tied to expressions of pleasure and enjoyment, and reflect the planned nature of determined drunkenness often found in sporting environments.

Although determined drunkenness in the context of sport carries particular connotations and expectations that return us to some of the assumptions about masculine behaviours the book is concerned to challenge, extreme drinking is by no means particular to sport. Hen and Stag nights, shore leave, university 'Fresher' or Orientation weeks, and school breaks, or simply 'big night outs' are among those occasions where deliberately drinking to excess is a key part of the occasion itself (Rosen, 1988; Lindsay, 2006; Carpenter, et al., 2008; Berwick, et al., 2008; Thurnell-Read, 2011a; 2012; Harrison, et al., 2011).

What these occasions have in common is that the sociality and commensality of the activity is central to the activity itself. Indeed, as Griffin, et al.'s (2009) research with young people in Britain makes clear, the 'passing out stories' in which the evening or drinking event is recreated by those who were there serve as a ritualised means of bonding among peers that is highly valued by the drinkers

---

2   For the uninitiated, 'skulling', also known as 'necking' is the practice of downing a drink, usually beer, without stopping. Boat races are a team version of this practice, with teams racing each other to see who can consume their drinks the fastest. Perhaps the most extreme example of determined drunkenness is that of the former Australian cricketer David Boon's record of drinking 52 cans of beer on a flight between Sydney and London when he was a member of the Australian cricket team in 1994.

involved. Here, the commensual aspects of drinking are celebrated, and in this respect extreme drinking comes to represent a form of fiesta drunkenness (Gordon, et al., 2012).

Importantly, many of these tales of passing out, having fun and losing control involve great creativity and imagination. Storytelling and narrating drinking episodes or 'big nights out' adds to the pleasure and enjoyment of sport-related drinking. Fuchs and Le Hénaff's (2013) account of the 'third quarter' or post-match drinking sessions enjoyed by male and female amateur rugby players in France describes the creative energy that goes into extreme drinking, where much forethought, planning, time and effort goes into preparing for a drinking session. Here, the anticipation of the drinking encounter is an integral part of the occasion. As Griffin, et al. (2009) note in their evocatively titled paper, 'Every time I do it I absolutely annihilate myself', much of the enjoyment of determined drunkenness lies as much in the anticipatory rituals of preparing for the big night out as it does in the night itself or the passing out stories told after the event. As Chrzan notes, 'alcohol stories have emotional meanings' (2013: 121).

My own research into alcohol consumption among fans of Australian Rules football also provides some examples of the creative work that can underpin sport-related drinking. As I have written about elsewhere (Palmer and Thompson, 2007; Palmer, 2009), a particular group of (male) fans known as 'the Grog Squad' are distinctive for the ways in which they re-imagine many aspects of popular culture to reflect the centrality of drinking to members of the group.

Witness the adaptation of the popular board game Monopoly that can be found on the Grog Squad's website (rocketrooster.com). Now known as 'Grogopoly' some of the rules include:

1. Go to The Taj – go directly to The Taj[3] – do not pass the pub – spend $200 on booze;
2. You have won 2nd prize in a beer sculling contest – collect $15;
3. Caught fighting on the hill or clubrooms – buy each player one beer;
4. Caught throwing up at the footy – return all grog squad merchandise;
5. Getting drunk and thrown out of the club – return to The Taj and buy everyone a beer;
6. Caught drink driving on the way back from Noarlunga [a rival team's oval] – miss two turns.

The example of 'Grogopoly', I suggest, also alerts us to the creative energy that characterises the maintenance of this very particular cultural identity. Much forethought, planning, time and effort goes into making banners and 'floggers' [pom poms], printing T-shirts (see Figure 2.1) and coming up with the pranks and practical jokes that are central to their distinctive style of spectatorship.

---

3   'The Taj' is the name of the beer stall at the club's home football ground.

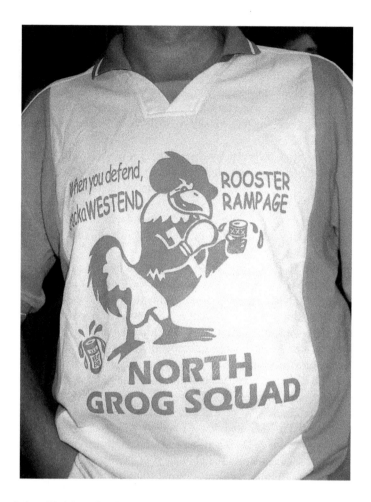

Figure 2.1   T-shirt of a Grog Squad member

Source: Photograph author's own

The rocketrooster.com website, for example, features a photo gallery of various banner and flogger making sessions which have taken place over the many years of the Grog Squad's existence while the account of the Grog Squad coming out to the centre of the football oval at half time to encircle the North Adelaide players (the team the Grog Squad follows) with a large sheet of black plastic when they were being resoundingly thrashed by their opponents has been elevated to the status of urban legend among the Grog Squad. The imagery is, of course, borrowed from horse racing, where a horse that is injured in a fall is covered in a black sheet before the race steward arrives to put it down out of public view.

The creativity associated with sport-related drinking can also be conceived as 'serious leisure' (Stebbins, 1997; 2001), whereby communities such as the Grog Squad provide opportunities for people to enact and embrace leisure-related activities that offer individuals ways and resources to distinguish themselves by developing specialised knowledge, skills and experiences. Spracklen (2013), for example, makes a similar observation in his ethnographic research on single-malt whisky enthusiasts, arguing that whisky enthusiasts are 'shaped by cultural capital about whisky' (2013: 56).

Writing about gun collectors and skydivers, Anderson and Taylor note that members of serious leisure communities 'may also feel marginalized when they perceive themselves and their activities as misunderstood by the broader society' (2010: 34). In much the same way, communities built explicitly around a culture of commitment to drinking to excess, such as that found with the Grog Squad, requires a negotiation of the boundaries between their leisure and other social institutions surrounding it and them.

Similarly, the 'Mad Monday' celebrations common in Australia that mark the end-of-season across the country's three dominant football codes can be thought of in this context. Sharing aspects of the carnivalesque; on the Monday after the Grand Final, players dress up, alcohol is consumed to excess, the social order is inverted and rules are transgressed (Hackley, et al., 2012). Activities and behaviours also skirt the boundaries of criminality. Witness the 2013 Mad Monday celebrations of one Australian Rules football club where a 'dwarf entertainer' who was hired as the occasion's 'entertainment' was set alight by a drunken player, yet no charges were laid (ABC, 2013).

While the serious leisure of extreme drinking and determined drunkenness can make the activity 'dammed fun' (Tutenges and Rod, 2009), it nonetheless remains problematic due to the quantities consumed, the activities that accompany the drinking, and the health and social impacts and consequences of the drinking. Here, we return to Brain's 'evident tension' (2009: 12) between the pursuit of pleasure and the discourses of self-care that emphasise moderation and restraint.

Distinction, Symbolic Capital and Sport-related Drinking

Studies of determined drunkenness also provide insight into studies of symbolic capital and the ways in which drinking, in the context of sport, acts as a symbolic marker of inclusion, belonging, status and prestige. It is here that the work of the French sociologist Pierre Bourdieu is particularly instructive.

Defined as 'the form that the various species of capital assume when they are perceived and recognized as legitimate' (Bourdieu, 1989: 17), symbolic capital can best be thought of as the resources available to an individual on the basis of honour, prestige or recognition which serve as the values held within a culture. Being able to 'drink well', for example, is an expression of a particular form of cultural competence among the Grog Squad. Erving Goffman once wrote – albeit in an entirely different context – that 'people are obliged not only to carry out their tasks and routines, but also *express* their competence in doing so' (1959: 33). For the Grog Squad, drinking competence is a key marker of cultural identity and it is through their regular, extended drinking sessions that they construct their personal reputations, as drinkers.

Bourdieu's (1989) work on symbolic capital and distinction has been usefully deployed elsewhere in drug and alcohol studies (Lunnay, et al., 2011), yet has not been systematically applied to an analysis of sport-related drinking. Lake's (2012) work on inclusion and exclusion in a competitive tennis club hints at the role of drinking in the exercise of symbolic and cultural capital, yet drinking is not the prime focus of his research. Similarly, Burdsey's research on the experiences of Muslim cricketers highlights the ways in which being non-drinkers excludes them from the accrual of particular forms of symbolic capital. While non-drinkers are discussed more fully in Chapter 4, the point here is that non-drinking underscores the ways in which drinking – either not doing it or doing too much of it – provides a key window on its capacity to demonstrate and mobilise symbolic capital in the context of sport.

The absence of a Bourdieusian perspective in studies of sport-related drinking specifically is surprising, given that much drinking is done for either social recognition or to achieve distinction or inclusion among one's sporting peers. Indeed, much of the research and scholarship notes that sport-related drinking is frequently done to achieve validation or recognition by fellow drinkers, yet the analytical point that is invariably made is that men drinking is marker of distinction among their male peers; that is, a display of hegemonic masculinity. While, prestige is defined and distinction is reasserted through drinking, full use has not been made of Bourdieu's concepts when explaining the social meaning of sport-related drinking. There is clearly more potential to applying Bourdieu's key concepts to analyses of drinking and sport, particularly when considering the symbolic capacity of drinking to establish and reinforce boundaries of distinction.

'Normalisation' Theory and Sport-related Drinking

Whilst not attributable to a single social theorist, the normalisation theory is 'one of the most influential recent developments in the sociology of drug use and has become something of an orthodoxy in the field' (Measham and Shiner, 2009: 502). In essence, the thesis contends that whereas illicit drug use in particular was once attributed to individual or social pathology, it has increasingly become a fairly unremarkable feature of young people's lives; now a 'part of the broader search for pleasure, excitement and enjoyment framed within consumption oriented leisure lifestyles' (Measham and Shiner, 2009: 502). In other words, it has moved 'from the margins to the centre of youth culture' (Parker, et al., 1998: 152). The idea of 'normalisation' also resonates with Gordon, et al.'s (2012) description of what they term 'banalized' drinking in which the consumption of alcohol is conceived as a routine rather than an exceptional social activity. For many, drinking at and because of sporting events is now an unremarkable feature of a broader cultural landscape.

While most commonly applied to studies of illegal drug use, aspects of the normalisation theory could usefully frame analyses of sport-related drinking. Certainly, the starting point for many studies of sport-related drinking is the premise that there is nothing remarkable about it. As Scott notes 'undoubtedly cultural conditions and accepted conventions determine where and how we drink. But who sets these conditions and conventions and how? For most of us, they just seem natural' (2001: 60–61). Yet, to be useful, theoretically, the obvious needs to be pushed a little further. What makes sport-related drinking unremarkable? Why is drinking considered to be 'just part of the culture'? What social, historical, political or other trends might account for the normalisation of sport-related drinking? Critically perhaps, is sport-related drinking 'normal' for all? That is, is normalisation a contingent process that is negotiated, accommodated or resisted by particular social groups operating in particular social situations? Or, put differently, where do the boundaries of 'normal' start and end in sport-related drinking? These are all potential avenues for further empirical research into the normalisation of sport-related drinking.

While the normalisation of sport-related drinking has largely occurred (along with the normalisation of gendered notions of hegemonic masculinity) at a societal level, researchers are finding that within individual sports and among pockets of particular sports fans, drinking has similarly become banalised; regarded as everyday and unexceptional. Again, my research with the Grog Squad is a useful case in point here. Reporting on a period of ethnographic research conducted with the 'Groggies', I describe how alcohol consumption is woven into the fabric of their interactions and identity, with regular drinking a way of conferring commitment and belonging to the group:

> among these exclusively male fans, heavy alcohol consumption is considered nothing untoward. Most weekends involve a substantial amount of drinking whilst watching the football, a proportion drink regularly throughout the week, and much attention is given over to preparing for the following weekend's drinking (Palmer, 2009: 225).

Such accounts of banalised drinking are useful analytically, in that they offer a way of considering the social context of drinking – the who, how and why of drinking – rather than the question of 'how much' which has typically occupied constructions of drinking typologies to date.

As I noted in the previous chapter, there has been a move away from questions of quantity to questions of experience; that is, what it felt like and what it meant to be drunk in a particular social situation. That the group of largely middle aged men who comprise the Grog Squad regard drinking as a routine cultural activity raises some questions about drinking, age, gender and the life-course. Mullen, et al. (2007), for example, argues that excessive drinking is presumed to be the preserve of young men. That is, as men age, they are perceived to 'grow out of it'. Similarly, women drinking to excess – in sport or elsewhere – provokes a wider social anxiety, whereby female drinkers are frequently portrayed as problematic, particularly in the news media (Measham and Østergaard, 2009), where the 'young drunken woman has become an archetypal symbol of the 'binge drinking' problem' (Atkinson, et al., 2012: 5). Both the public drinking of older men and drinking by women disrupt many of our taken-for-granted assumptions, yet more and more so, banalised drinking, particularly routinely drinking to excess, is becoming the rule rather than the exception to it. Further research is needed into the social and health costs and consequences of the banalisation of drinking, in sport or elsewhere. Here, questions of context are important for they situate actions within a particular setting or milieu that elsewhere may be considered problematic.

Writing about female participation in street gangs, Messerschmidt (1995) makes the point that what may seem abnormal or out of place in one context makes sense in terms of broader social structures in another context:

> what is usually considered atypical feminine behaviour outside of the situation is, in fact, *normalized* within the social context of inner-neighbourhood conflict: girl gang violence in this situation is encouraged, permitted and privileged by *both* boys and girls as appropriate feminine behaviour. Thus 'bad girl' femininity is situationally accomplished and context bound within the domain of the street (1995: 182, original emphasis).

Following Messerschmidt, an exploration of the ways in which people 'do drinking' in relation to sport allows us to ask questions of the context or the 'definitions of the situation' (Thomas, 1937 in Herman-Kinney and Kinney, 2012: 4) that have made it so very unremarkable.

Foucault, Sport and Alcohol

The banalisation or normalisation of drinking – in sport or elsewhere – has downplayed the role of structural influences, emphasising instead the rational actions of individuals in understanding their alcohol use. Certainly, the conscious decision to drink in particular ways and contexts suggests a high degree of agency among drinking groups like the Grog Squad. Yet agency operates in concert with structure, and the work of Michel Foucault focuses on the ways in which individual subjects – in this case drinkers – are caught between governing the self; that is exercising agency or self-control and being governed by the other; that is, by governmental policies and practices such as taxes, levies and regulation by and of the alcohol industry. As Hacking writes:

> we are all "made up" through a combination of the categories and labels asserted 'from above" and the "autonomous behaviour of the person so labelled, which

presses from below. These processes shape both "what we are" and also "the possibilities for what we might have been" (1986: 233).

In analyses of drug and alcohol policy in particular, Foucault's concepts of disciplinary power, biopower and governmentality are frequently used to explain the social construction of drugs and alcohol as a 'problem', how to treat drug users and how drug users and addicts are constructed and positioned as medico-legal subjects (Bourgois, 2000; Keane, 2009; Duff; 2008). From Foucault's work on sexuality, imprisonment and mental health, we recognise that power circulates among people, continually produced and reproduced in their discourse and practices, allowing drugs and alcohol to be studied in the contexts in which they are produced, governed, traded and used (Bourgois, 2000).

By way of illustration, Thompson, et al.'s (2007) analysis of anti-smoking and smoking cessation programmes in New Zealand suggests that conventional methods of health promotion may be ignored or prompt resistance rather than compliance on the part of the individuals being targeted in smoking awareness campaigns and parallels can certainly be drawn in relation to alcohol awareness, the responsible consumption of alcohol, and the resistance to such campaigns, which are discussed further in Chapters 6 and 8. Further, Thompson, et al. (2007) suggests that anti-smoking policies may compound existing inequalities. Those who continue to smoke tend to be clustered in socio-economically deprived areas that are themselves stigmatised and within these areas poor smokers can be subject to dual stigmatisation, thus highlighting the uneven workings of biopower.

Accordingly, while being cast as an 'outsider' may stimulate behaviour change, it may equally give rise to active resistance. The analysis can be extended to the stigma attached to drinking places and locational disadvantage, and resistance to health-promotion strategies as they relate to alcohol consumption, and this theme is explored further in Chapter 8. For the moment however, such examples underscore the interplay between structure and agency and the potential of sociological models to help us characterise and understand some of the complex interactions that bind sport and alcohol in particular ways.

Following on from this, a key focus of the 'new public health' (Baum, 2008) is that individuals should learn to know their own limits, be that in terms of diet, exercise, smoking or alcohol use. Monitoring or self-regulating one's drinking thus involves reflecting on how a person might behave in relation to the regulatory and policing measures designed to protect them; that is, to resist or comply. In other words, public health initiatives such as alcohol harm minimisation campaigns operate as a form of governance 'at a distance' (Rose and Miller, 1992: 184–6), whereby the notion of public health or health for all is constituted out of a combination of techniques and strategies that involve the relations between people and the structures and institutions within which these strategies and relationships sit (Foucault, 1991).

So, what then, might a Foucaldian analysis of sport-related drinking look like? Certainly, Foucault's focus on disciplinary power and governmentality can help us to move beyond understanding subjectivities and peoples' experiences of sport-related drinking (which Bourdieu's work on symbolic capital and the normalisation theory allow us to do) to looking at networks of governance in which drinkers become regulated subjects, or at the decisions, interactions and consequences of sport-related drinking that form part of a broader 'risk discourse' that underscores wider debates about individual choice, agency, structure and context. These are preliminary possibilities that lay the foundation for a more developed, explicitly Foucauldian, research agenda around sport and alcohol.

Risk and Pleasure

The ideas and theories of Foucault and Bourdieu serve, in different ways, to highlight a fundamental tension in writing about sport and alcohol and, indeed, alcohol consumption more broadly, namely the tension between the regulation or mitigation of risk and ideas of pleasure and enjoyment. Writing about young people's experimentation with drug and alcohol use, Järvinen and Østergaard note that 'the relationship of young people to drugs is influenced not just by their risk perceptions and risk willingness, but also by the pleasure and excitement they associate with drug use' (2011: 334). Indeed, while contemporary drug and alcohol policies largely advocate harm minimisation and 'doing things a little less dangerously', the sheer pleasure and enjoyment of alcohol intoxication operates as a considerable barrier to policy uptake and compliance, for it represents the antithesis to many of the assumptions of moderation, regulation and self-control which underpin dominant policy approaches to alcohol misuse. In other words, while the pleasure of intoxication may not be considered 'warrantable motives' for consumption by policy and lawmakers (O'Malley and Valverde, 2004), it is precisely in this fashion that much sport-related drinking is done, and needs to be considered as an integral part of the wider policy discourse and debate.

The idea of 'pleasure' has much currency in sport and leisure studies more broadly, and researchers have been attentive to notions of enjoyment, thrill seeking and hedonism in activities like skydiving and snowboarding where concepts such as 'edgework' are an integral part of the discourse (Lyng, 1990; 2005; Laurendreau, 2008; Thorpe, 2012). It is not my intention to rehearse those themes and debates here. Rather, my concern is to extend the discussion of the centrality of pleasure in sport to a discussion of the absence of pleasure when considering the *policy* implications of sports-associated drinking in the context of the theoretical frameworks introduced earlier.

While these debates are picked up again in Chapter 8, the pleasure of intoxication, its absence in critical discourse and the challenges it presents for policy formulation is by no means a new debate in studies of *illicit* drug and alcohol use, particularly by young people (Measham, et al., 2001; Coveney and Bunton, 2003; Moore, 2008; Dwyer, 2008; Duff, 2008; Zajdow, 2010; Järvinen and Østergaard, 2011), where scholars have drawn attention to the 'preoccupation of earlier research with risk awareness and (especially) risk-unawareness among young people and for ignoring the positive expectations and experiences youths have in relation to drugs' (Järvinen and Østergaard, 2011: 334). The debate about pleasure, as either celebrated, denied or problematised, is, however, yet to register in discussions of policy that relate to drugs and alcohol *in sport*, and this is my central concern here.

While researchers have observed for some time how pleasure is bound to social context, there is a need to consider what Duff (2008) describes as 'pleasure practice'; the lived experiences of drinkers, in this case, for the enjoyable physical effects of alcohol can, in some cases, enrich activities like 'dancing, social interaction, conversation, sex and so on' (Duff, 2008: 387) and the sensory dimensions of drinking are inextricably linked to the social and cultural settings in which alcohol is consumed which, in turn, sets boundaries and limits around public health policy and strategy in particular ways.

Public health strategies are typically based on a concordance model that seeks to persuade individuals to minimise harm to themselves and others through 'low risk' drinking. Harrison, et al. (2011) in their review of the Australian government's efforts to control the consumption of alcohol argue that such strategies are limited and unlikely to achieve the desired effect. In particular, they note that these strategies define young people in a particular way; ascribing a particular rationality to the choices young people make about their drinking.

Similarly, Hayward and Hobbs (2007) point to what they describe as a wider dialectic surrounding contemporary 'binge drinking', and in particular the relationship between aesthetic processes aimed at encouraging alcohol-related excitement and excess (i.e. alcohol's promotional culture), and those that seek to exert a measure of rational control over the 'problem' of excessive alcohol consumption. As Alaszewski notes, research on alcohol and risk as 'focussed either on the ways in which governments try and manage the risks associated with drugs or on the ways in which individuals perceive the risks associated with drugs and how this influences patterns of use' (2011: 390), means that regulators do not consider the perceived benefits and pleasures of drug-taking or consuming alcohol. In much the same way, Crichter (2011) argues that the moral regulation of alcohol consumption is integral to wider processes of moral regulation that centre on the question of what is and what is not legitimate pleasure.

In positioning sport-related drinking as a form of 'calculated hedonism' or a resource through which to demonstrate one's symbolic capital, the problem of pleasure is also introduced as a major barrier to uptake and compliance with a number of policies and strategies designed to minimise the harms and risks associated with sport-related drinking. Notions of calculated hedonism and determined drunkenness present club officials, governing bodies and policy makers with a dilemma, for it clashes with other expectations of citizens, including notions of responsibility, reasonableness and self-control. Thinking about the politics of pleasure that underpin determined drunkenness and calculated hedonism allow us to enter into a broader debate about self-control, contradictory messages in alcohol advertising about 'having fun' and the normalisation of particular kinds of drinking – and drinkers – in sport.

The normalisation of drinking to excess – and the potential harms associated with it – runs counter to the risk discourse that dominates policy debates. For young people, in particular, the risk of injury, or even death, is often very far from their thoughts when engaged in a drinking encounter or associated behaviours. Nygaard, et al. (2003), for example, interviewed young people in Norway who had been involved in drink driving episodes about their experiences of driving while under the influence and/or riding with drunk drivers. They found that while substance-impaired driving increased the crash risks for young novice drivers who were more likely to speed, make errors and carry passengers in risky circumstances thereby placing themselves, their passengers, and other road users at greater risk of injury and death, the occupants of the car *at the time* considered that moment to be one of great thrill and an adrenalin rush.

Similar arguments have been made in relation to voluntary risk-taking through 'dangerous' lifestyle choices and decisions. In their evocatively titled paper: 'Life would be pretty dull without risk', Lupton and Tulloch (2002) maintain that voluntary risk-taking has its own particular pleasures that cannot be denied. Drug-taking, driving fast cars, having unprotected sex and taking part in extreme sports are amongst the 'pleasure pursuits' that Lupton and Tulloch identify, suggesting that experiences of risk are selfish and hedonic; risk seeking is about satisfying personal urges and desires, a view that sits in opposition to the de-personalised interpretation of risk popularly espoused by the German sociologist Ulrich Beck (1992). Drawing on the theoretical basis of Douglas (1966; 1992) and Douglas and Wildavsky (1982), this cultural approach to risk suggests that responses to risk, threat and uncertainty are done in prescribed ways that serve to maintain the boundaries and membership of particular groups and organisations (Le Breton, 2000; Palmer, 2004).

While there is a danger, perhaps, in the language of 'determined drunkenness', 'fiesta drunkenness' or 'extreme drinking' of celebrating or valorising risk and drinking to excess – in sport or elsewhere – recognising that the fun and pleasure of drinking are legitimate sources of meaning does not detract from broader issues relating to health, social policy, governance and regulation. Indeed, the tensions and challenges inherent in the pleasure of drinking cannot be simply glossed in the language of camaraderie and sociality that 'determined drunkenness', fiesta drunkenness or extreme drinking suggests.

What notions such as 'determined drunkenness' or 'extreme drinking' do, however, is suggest is that particular kinds of drinking practices have captured our attention analytically, with excessive drinking, more often than not, occupying much of the space in critical research and scholarship. It is here, I suggest, that there is a need to open up the theoretical terrain within which drinking, particularly sport-related drinking, has been conceptualised. As I elaborate in the following section, extreme drinking or determined drunkenness operates as a form of hegemonic drinking in which drinking, as a 'state or condition of ideology frames understandings of how particular ways of performing drinking are seen as natural and normal' (Palmer, 2013a: 5).

Towards Hegemonic Drinking?

The conceptualisation of 'hegemonic drinking', is, in some ways, little more than the normalisation of the expectation that heavy, problematic, drinking is an integral part of sporting identities, cultures and practices. As Thompson, Palmer and Raven note 'when drinking has been explored as part of the social world of [Australian Rules] football fans it has generally been in terms of excessive and irresponsible alcohol consumption' (2011: 390). With 'determined drunkenness' constructed, presented and expected as the dominant archetype for sport-related drinking, it becomes a hegemonic practice, carrying with it a particular kind of drinking 'capital' which is produced and reproduced through the exercise, embodiment and enactment of a certain kind of drinking mastery.

Inasmuch as hegemonic masculinity is the exercise and accrual of gender capital, hegemonic drinking operates in similar ways. In hegemonic drinking, 'dominant, powerful practices and tropes' (Palmer, 2013a: 5) operate in which the drinker is expected to be able to drink, and to drink well, or to demonstrate drinking competence. As Peralta notes, it is possible to 'upgrade' masculine capital through consuming and tolerating alcohol (2007: x), but this needs to be done in particular, culturally prescribed ways, and this is where the 'power' of drinking resides. Although hegemonic masculinity may be, as suggested earlier, fluid, it nonetheless continues to exist as both the source and the demonstration of *symbolic* capital. In much the same way, hegemonic drinking – drinking heavily, with all that entails – operates as both the source and the demonstration of symbolic capital in the context of a range of sporting codes and competitions. Moreover, it is the ways in which excessive drinking continues to dominate the discourse, analysis and policy agenda that contributes much to its hegemonic power.

Conclusion

This chapter has sketched out four alternative theoretical frameworks for explaining sport-related drinking. My starting point was that established concepts such as 'hegemonic masculinity' have much to offer, however they need to be reworked and reframed in light of continuing changes in patterns of alcohol consumption. My central argument has been that social scientists with an interest in drinking more broadly have been more attentive to other theoretical frameworks when explaining the cultural practices, social interactions and, indeed, consequences, of consuming alcohol, and drawing on these may lead to a more nuanced or developed understanding of sport-related drinking.

While I presented these as four relatively discrete ways in which people engage with alcohol in sporting contexts, this has been done for reasons of analytical simplicity. The schema is not always as clear cut as is suggested here; the theories, the assumptions that underpin them and the drinking practices they are intended to capture may overlap at different times and in different contexts. The expanded theoretical repertoire does, however, recognise the complexity of drinkers and drinking in sport, and helps to move the research agenda beyond the default theoretical position of equating sport-related drinking with notions of hegemonic masculinity. While drinking (and sport) certainly exist as sites and activities through which a particular, archetypical form of masculinity can be enacted, the idea of hegemonic masculinity alone does not capture the range of social actors and practices involved with sport-related drinking, nor the complex, interwoven and often contradictory issues that surround the sport-alcohol nexus.

While my concern here was with the limited ways in which sport-related drinking has been theorised and problematised, and risk glossing (or missing) critical questions for understanding alcohol use, in the process. Other behaviours and practices deemed to be 'unhealthy' have similarly been treated through a default theoretical, conceptual and at times moral standpoint. Writing about the dominant obesity discourse, for example, Mansfield and Rich note that:

> as scholars who have been involved with a growing community who are critical of the overbearing emphasis on obesity and overweight within health policy and practice we are concerned about the tendency in some quarters towards the deconstruction of dominant obesity discourse without offering some deliberations on how we might move the field of physical activity forward (2013: 1).

In the same way that Mansfield and Rich maintain that it is not enough to simply offer a critique without providing an alternative, conceptualising sport-related drinking through a number of alternative conceptual framings is a useful way of advancing the debate from one focused on hegemonic masculinity to one that acknowledges a number of ways in which sports consumption and alcohol consumption come together, for it considers the ways in which competing and underrepresented views (those of women and non-drinkers, discussed in the following chapters, for example) might be included in broader debates about the cultures and consequences of sport-related drinking.

Although I have outlined the ways in which four additional theoretical frameworks may be applied to studies of sport-related drinking, these of course need data and analysis to turn them from the abstract to the concrete, and the next two chapters, in particular, provide case studies drawn from empirical data to bring the argument to life. I've made the point elsewhere that there is a need for a 'more inclusive suite of methods to tease out some of the more nuanced understandings of the relationships between sport consumers and alcohol ... through ethnography, visual methods, focus groups, interviews or surveys' (Palmer, 2011: 179), and much of this book makes use of a broader sweep of methods to those that are customarily adopted in studies of sport and alcohol. Moving beyond hegemonic masculinity, the following chapter draws on empirical, qualitative research to explore the ways in which women understand and articulate their experiences of sport-related drinking, as consumers and in the context of Foucault's (1988) notion of 'care of self' and care of others.

Chapter 3

Women and Sport-related Drinking

This chapter:
- examines women and sport-related drinking;
- focuses on the experiences and understandings of sport-related drinking as articulated by female followers of Australian Rules football;
- offers some reflections on the politics and pragmatic realties of female researchers working in predominantly male research environments.

Introduction

One of the key concerns of the book is with the gaps and silences in what has been written about drinking and sport. In the previous chapter, I was critical of the seeming failure or reluctance of analyses of sport-related drinking to move beyond the argument that links the consumption of alcohol with assertions of 'hegemonic masculinity', and I argued that sociological accounts of sport-related drinking, in particular, have relied on fairly limited and predictable theoretical perspectives through which to frame their analyses. I suggested that social scientists with an interest in drinking more broadly have seen the possibilities of other theoretical frameworks for explaining the cultural practices, social interactions and, indeed, the consequences of consuming alcohol. For those of us with an interest in the consumption of sport as well as the consumption of alcohol, drawing on perspectives such as 'calculated hedonism', 'symbolic capital', 'serious leisure', 'governmentality', 'biopower' and the normalisation or banalisation of drinking may lead to a more nuanced and sophisticated understanding of sport-related drinking.

Tracing out these other theoretical possibilities through which we might approach the complex and at times contradictory range of social actors and drinking practices within the sport-alcohol nexus also started to hint at the idea that there are *new* relationships emerging between sport and alcohol, which also begin to question the dominance of hegemonic masculinity as a conceptual framework. Female drinkers, non-drinkers and light or social drinkers, drinkers in alternative and lifestyle sport or in sporting settings that are counter-intuitive to the sport-alcohol nexus (such as lawn bowls, yachting or Ultimate Frisbee, among others), as well as older men, gay men, non-Anglo men and other males who sit outside of normative assumptions of men in sport are playing a growing role in the sport-alcohol nexus, yet these remain under-researched and under-theorised.

With this as background, the focus of this chapter is on just one of these under-explored areas; namely women and sport-related drinking. Its concerns are two-fold. The chapter looks, firstly at the experiences and understandings of sport-related drinking as articulated by female followers of Australian Rules football. It then offers some reflections on my own experiences as a female researcher working in a predominantly male research environment. While the empirical context is that of Australian football, the material discussed in the chapter and the questions it raises are of broader relevance to a range of sporting settings in which alcohol is crucially implicated and where female researchers need to negotiate the subtle and not-so-subtle politics and pragmatic realities of their research environment.

Readers may perhaps expect a discussion of the role of alcohol in perpetuating sexual and other forms of violence against women, given the focus of the chapter on women and sport-related drinking. This is not an emphasis in this chapter and the issue is addressed more substantively in Chapter 8. The concerns of this chapter are far more with the role of alcohol in constructing and maintaining personal and social identities for women in a particular sporting setting, and the particular definitions and understandings that women may ascribe to sport-related drinking.

The chapter unfolds as follows: it begins by considering existing research on alcohol and gender, before moving to a discussion of the broader research on women and drinking, in which women are implicated in a discourse of problematic 'binge' drinking, risk and regulation. This provides the starting point from which to introduce the empirical detail that informs the rest of the chapter. Here, three gaps are underscored: i) the relative absence of discussion on *women* in the literature on sport, alcohol and gender; ii) the relative absence of *drinking* when considering female sporting identities and practices; and iii) the relative absence of *sport* in a discussion of female drinking in a broader social context. Although 'the relationship between gender and drug use remains the big neglected question in the field of substance use' (Measham, 2003: 22), the omission is not gender *per se* – men's relationship to and experiences of alcohol are well documented – but the relative absence of women in this literature as it relates, particularly, to sport. The chapter then concludes with a reflection on my experiences as a female researcher conducting research in a largely male environment.

Gender and Alcohol[1]

Despite the complex and contradictory relationship between gender and alcohol, previous studies have tended to focus on dichotomous differences between male and female drinking, particularly in terms of quantity and consequences. As

---

1   Parts of this section have been previously published in C. Palmer (2013b) Drinking like a guy? Women and sport related drinking. *Journal of Gender Studies*, 1–13.

Borgen notes 'the dominant approach to gender in alcohol research still conceives of gender in terms of binary roles and looks for explanations for gender differences in drinking' (2011: 155). Research into alcohol-related behaviour consistently finds that 'men outnumber women as alcohol consumers, drink greater quantities of alcohol and experience more health and social problems as a consequence of their alcohol use' (Atkinson, Kirton and Summall, 2012: 5). In these gender-focussed analyses of alcohol and other drug use, the emphasis has usually been on the individual male or female or on the genders as aggregates of the individuals. Thus, there is a considerable focus in the literature as to whether heavy drinking among women has increased or whether male and female rates of heavy drinking have converged (Bloomfield, et al., 2001; Holmila and Raitasalo, 2005), yet far less has focussed on the social meanings and cultural practices that surround the rates or levels of consumption either by women or by men (or other women) as understood by women. This is the concern of what follows.

Much of the research on gender differences into prevalence and quantity of alcohol consumption in relation to sport has been undertaken with specific cohorts. College students, particularly student athletes and sports sciences students from Northern America and Europe universities are widely studied groups, with the extant literature focussing on their socio-demographic characteristics and their self-reported alcohol use (Gill, 2002; Ford, 2007; Peralta and Steel, 2009; Peralta, et al., 2010; Maggs, Rankin and Lee, 2011; De Vissesr and McDonnell, 2012). The consistent finding is that male students are more likely to drink, and drink at high levels, than their female counterparts (Peralta, et al., 2010). Both men and women, however, report a range of negative consequences of their drinking such as drunk driving, injuries and fatalities, encounters with the legal system, and sexual and physical violence, as well as certain benefits such as the camaraderie and social networks accrued by participating in the 'party' scene, particularly the drinking games and activities that are a frequent part of college life (Caparo, 2000; Tutenges and Sandberg, 2013).

While it is an issue to which I will return shortly, the point to note from such comparative studies of male and female drinking is that studies of *all female* drinking groups are rare. Honkassalo's (1989) participant-observation study of drinking parties among Finnish female factory workers is one of the rare examples, and is an important contribution to the literature in that it privileges the experiences and understandings of the social meanings of drinking as a cultural practice among women, rather than it being relative to the experience of men or, alternatively, as understood through a lens of resistance to normative expectations of femininity and/or a particular class habitus – common analytical devices in studies of drinking by women. Much of this literature that expands on these themes is reviewed in what follows.

Alongside the quantitative data which presents patterns of difference between men's and women's drinking among discrete population cohorts, several qualitative studies highlight how alcohol is significant in young people's constructions of social identity, where peer drinking is an immensely pleasurable (albeit problematic) pastime. As I suggested in the previous chapter, drinking to excess has its own pleasures that cannot be denied. At the same time, there is a tension between perceptions of risk and the possibilities of dangers and the fun and enjoyment of determined drunkenness that equally cannot be ignored. The important point for this chapter is that many of the tales of passing out, having fun and losing control that are central to fiesta drunkenness or calculated hedonism have been 'condoned and encouraged within the strictures of hegemonic masculinity' (Thurnell-Read, 2011a: 978); that is, they have come to occupy a place within the popular (and sociological) imagination as forms of male behaviour, more particularly the expression of *hegemonic* masculinity; that is, the culturally normative form of male behaviour which subordinates femininity and other forms of masculinity, such as ageing men or gay men that I discussed in the previous chapter.

Of concern in this chapter, the over-reliance on a discourse of hegemonic masculinity to frame the 'doing' of drinking and the imaginative work that often accompanies it raises a series of questions. What about female drinking in sport? Does 'hegemonic masculinity' still have analytical utility when women are the subjects of study? If not, then what alternative theoretical frameworks could be applied as well? Are any of the theoretical frameworks introduced in the previous chapter better for understanding women and sport-related drinking? There is also a semi-rhetorical question here that speaks to a broader feminist critique of sport that raises concerns of power, privilege, exclusion, gaps and silences. Why has female drinking in sport largely eluded sociological inquiry, and what new (or recurrent) themes and issues for studies of alcohol, identity, gender and social relationships may be raised by studies of female drinking and sport? These themes and questions are addressed in the ensuing pages.

Women and Alcohol

Although men, statistically, consume greater quantities of alcohol than women, there has 'in recent years been a marked increase in alcohol consumption by young women in Western countries' (Lyons and Willott, 2008: 694). Such changes in drinking patterns has led to a wider social anxiety with 'binge' drinking and public drinking, whereby female drinkers are frequently portrayed as problematic, particularly in the news media (Measham and Østergaard, 2009), where the 'young drunken woman has become an archetypal symbol of the "binge drinking" problem' (Atkinson, et al., 2012: 5).

At the same time, whilst often portrayed as 'at risk' from predatory men, female drinkers are frequently depicted as lacking in femininity (Jackson and Tinkler, 2007; Griffin, et al., 2009) or conversely, as sexually promiscuous or enacting an 'emphasized femininity' (Connell, 1987), in which they dress and act to accommodate male interests. In her studies of hen nights in Britain, for example, Skeggs (1997; 2005) notes that the women involved in these female only, pre-wedding drinking occasions exhibit a preoccupation with beauty, flirtatiousness and sexual availability that re-inscribes heteronormativity in very particular, very public ways.

As I address in the empirical details that follow, while women who engage in and enact such behaviours may be stigmatised and subject to a particular kind of (class-based) moral scrutiny far more readily than men who are 'off the leash and out of control' (Thurnell-Read, 2011a), for the female fans of Australia Rules football who's drinking experiences inform this chapter, such experiences are seen as a legitimate cultural space in which their identities as sporting fans and supporters are played out through competing discourses of responsibility, restraint, enjoyment and pleasure. Relative to the work done on male drinking, in sport or elsewhere, very few studies have examined the meanings and social contexts of women's drinking, and it is this gap in the research that this chapter seeks to address.

Given the wider discursive construction of female drinking as problematic, it is perhaps not surprising that women's drinking has rarely been regarded as pleasurable, but, instead, almost exclusively, in wholly negative terms. As Measham notes, 'the broad characterization unfolds in one of two ways: women's lives are worse than men's and therefore they take drugs and use alcohol to make their lives better or, for younger women in particular recreational/celebratory that is bound up in a discourse of risk taking' (2003: 22).

To push this line of argument further, the first of these narratives of women's drug and alcohol use unfolds as 'problematic', in which usage is linked to the depiction of women self-medicating for relief from poverty, depression and desperation, leading to entrapment in in petty acquisitive crime and sex work to pay for their drugs (Measham, 2003: 22). The second, contrasting, narrative focuses on recreational drug and alcohol use, in which women's lives are perceived as mirroring men's lives in a variety of spheres, such as increased education and employment opportunities.[2] Of concern here, there is a focus on converging consumption patterns around legal and illicit drug use, whereby women are seen to take on the behaviours of men in relation to leisure pursuits, in which drugs and alcohol play an integral part. This is epitomised in the 'work hard, play hard "ladette" culture much loved by the media, which evokes swarms of young, single and "up for it" party girls besieging the café bar cities of the Western world' (Measham, 2003: 2).

Neither of these stereotypes is particularly useful for or illuminating of alcohol use or the complexities of women's lives in relation to sports-associated drinking. As is evident from the empirical research described in the following pages, women's relationships to sport-related drinking are both complex and contradictory, with narratives of responsibility, restraint, pleasure and enjoyment all being part of a collective discourse of what I described in the previous chapter and elsewhere (Palmer, 2013a; Palmer, 2013b) as 'hegemonic drinking' (rather than hegemonic masculinity) in which particular drinking practices occupy positions of social and

---

2 Room also suggests that eight specific aspects of gender roles should be considered when exploring women's experiences of alcohol: courtship and affectional preference, sexuality, marriage and partnership, parenthood friendship and peer relations, work roles, informal social control and domination, violence and crime (1996: 228).

symbolic pre-eminence. Rather than see sport-related drinking as an enactment of masculinity or a transgression of femininity (the 'go-to' explanations for drinking by men and women) I argue that to explain drinking practices simply in terms of conformity and resistance to gender role socialisation is to obscure the ways in which women 'do drinking' and the contributions this may make to studies of sports-related drinking, the sociality of alcohol consumption and the sociology of sport and gender studies more broadly.

While Measham's (2003) depiction of women self-medicating for relief from poverty, depression and desperation certainly has some relevance for women and sport-related drinking, this was not evidenced in the data described shortly. This is not to suggest that sportswomen do not experience problematic relationships to alcohol – biographical accounts from several high profile sportswomen who have battled with alcohol addictions tell a different story[3] and are part of the sport-alcohol nexus that I describe in Chapter 5 – however, the experiences of female Australian sports fans suggests a more nuanced relationship to alcohol and sport than the blunt theoretical tools and conceptual frameworks have hitherto allowed.

What About Sport?

To return now to sport-related drinking, it is noteworthy that studies of alcohol and sport have mirrored the emphases and omissions in accounts of gender and alcohol more broadly. Men have been the emphasis, and hegemonic masculinity deployed as the dominant theoretical paradigm for conceptualising men's sport-related drinking. As I discussed in the previous chapter, while the sociology of sport has made a considerable contribution to studies of the ways in which alcohol plays an important role in creating particular cultural identities, this has been done, almost exclusively, in relation to masculine identities.

There are two notable exceptions that provide a useful complement to my research with female followers of sport rather than female participants. Fuchs and Le Hénaff's (2013) ethnographic research with a women's rugby team in France argues that far from being only a male preserve, the 'third half-time' (a colloquialism for post-match festivities) and its related drinking activities are also done by women who, for their part, use a similar narrative or rhetoric to evoke the meanings attached to post-match drinking practices. Echoing my earlier observation that very few studies in the literature address alcohol consumption by sportswomen, Fuchs and Le Hénaff (2013) argue that this type of drinking has a specific meaning in which drinking by women is both normative and threatening or transgressive at one and the same time.

---

3   See, for example, *Footballer: My Story* – the autobiography of Kelly Smith, the captain of the English women's football squad, or *Riding Wild*, the autobiography of former Australian surfing champion, Pam Buridge, both of which document the author's battles with alcohol addictions.

Similarly, Litchfield and Diongi's (2012) work with a female veterans' field hockey team in Australia explores the importance of drinking rituals among an ageing (well, 45 years and over!), yet highly competitive team. Drawing on in-depth interviews and field observations undertaken during matches and a tournament championship dinner, Litchfield and Diongi (2012) argue that drinking is a recurring ritual that was woven into the cultural expectations and experiences of this group of sportswomen. Practical jokes, comedic team mascots and uniforms, along with the sharing of a drink after matches allowed for social connections, enjoyment and feelings of empowerment that extended beyond just playing hockey. While Fuchs and Le Hénaff's (2013) and Litchfield and Diongi's (2012) work is illustrative of the possibilities for analyses of women and sport-related drinking, accounts of the sociality of sport-related drinking as told by women remain few and far between, and it is an account of the social context or the 'definitions of the situation' (Thomas, 1937 in Herman-Kinney and Kinney, 2012: 4) in which drinking by female sports fans occurs that is explored in the following pages.

The lack of research on female drinking and sport is both striking and surprising, given on-going concerns with female drinking more widely, and its location within a discourse of risk, responsibility and 'appropriate' female behaviours when drinking, particularly drinking in public, as this tends to be the space in which sport-related drinking occurs – at sporting grounds, venues, pubs and clubs, and the like. To offer something of a counter to the limitations sketched so far, the paper turns now to the empirical research with female fans of Australian Rules football, and their experiences and understandings of their own and other's alcohol consumption.

A Note on Methodology

The data and initial impetus for this chapter came from a period of ethnographic fieldwork undertaken throughout the 2005 season of the South Australian National Football League [SANFL] as part of a broader project on the social meanings of alcohol in Australian football.[4] Data were collected from participant-observation undertaken in metropolitan Adelaide (the capital of South Australia and the fifth largest Australian capital city) between March and October. Fieldwork was conducted with nine football clubs at 25 games over the season including the preliminary and grand finals. Two female researchers attended football matches, visiting football grounds, clubrooms, bistros and bars, and a variety of social functions such as pre-game sponsors' lunches, after game presentations, bingo days, 'Claret and Stout' lunches and members' happy hours.

---

4 The SANFL refers to the South Australian National Football League, a state-based second tier league to the national Australian Football League. The methods and methodological concerns this study raised have been more fully detailed in Palmer and Thompson (2007; 2010).

To contextualise the findings from the participant-observation, semi-structured, open-ended interviews were conducted with 93 participants; 67 men and 26 women from across the nine SANFL clubs whose membership represented the broad demographic base of suburban Adelaide. It is the interviews with the women that provide the data for this chapter.[5]

Participants

Twenty-six women aged 25 to 86 were interviewed from across the nine clubs. The women were recruited for voluntary participation using flyers distributed at football grounds and through club-based newsletters, and all were unknown to the researchers. Participants were all white, Anglo-Australian, and all were in heterosexual relationships. Eighteen of the women were mothers, two were grandmothers, and the women held a range of professional occupations, including teachers, nurses, lawyers, an academic, and tertiary students, as well as three retirees.

As self-defined 'fans' of any one of the nine teams who played in the South Australian National Football league, the women interviewed were frequent, visible and vocal fixtures at each week's game, and many had long associations with a club, having supported their team since their childhood.[6] Fourteen of the women occupied some kind of volunteer role within their club, serving as club secretary, treasurer, 'uniforms officer', 'strapper', 'chief bar maid' or 'head of the canteen', among others.

Procedures

The interviews, which lasted for approximately 45–60 minutes, were conducted in respondents' own homes. As well as helping to triangulate the data collected at football grounds and venues, the interviews provided first-hand accounts of the women's experiences and understandings of their own and others' alcohol consumption in particular sporting settings. While the topic of discussion was sport-related drinking, alcohol was not consumed by the participants or the researchers during the interviews (a debate I return to in Chapter 9), although the women all indicated that they consumed alcohol as part of their routine experiences of following football.[7]

---

5   The sample of 67 (72 per cent) male interviewees was representative of SANFL records, which indicated that 72 per cent of club members were male.

6   While definitions of 'fan', the relative absence of women in discussions of fan culture, and how one becomes a fan or expresses their fan identity or allegiance are all subjects of critical scrutiny (Crawford, 2004; Pope, 2011; Mewett and Toffoletti, 2011; Toffoletti and Mewett, 2012), such processes of becoming and belonging are less central to this paper and its focus on women's experiences and understandings of their own and others sport-related drinking.

7   Although alcohol was not consumed during the interviews it was, at times, consumed when participants attended football matches and after game functions. The ethical and reflexive dimensions of doing this (and other) research where alcohol was consumed have been documented more fully in Palmer and Thompson (2010).

The interviews were digitally recorded, transcribed and coded independently by two female researchers using an agreed upon template to ensure consistency of data recording across the project. As noted elsewhere, 'having two researchers enabled us to triangulate key themes emerging from the data and to double check any gaps in our field notes, ensuring rigour in the write up and subsequent analysis of this material' (Palmer and Thompson, 2007: 191). The interview data were thematically analysed with the assistance of the NVIVO software package, using a 'constant-comparative' method of emerging themes' similarly employed by Anderson, McCormack and Lee (2012). The research was conducted in compliance with the Australian National Health and Medical Research Council's Ethical Guidelines, in which informed consent was obtained prior to participation in the interviews, the right to withdraw from the research respected, and the identities of research participants protected, with pseudonyms adopted for the reporting of data.

Key Themes

Responsibility and restraint
The long-standing association that participants had with a football club mediated their relationship to alcohol and shaped it in particular ways. As mentioned earlier, many women held volunteer positions within a club, and these unpaid roles meant they often had a position of responsibility with regard to the serving of alcohol and the monitoring of its use, both formally and informally. The longevity of involvement with a football club meant that these women frequently 'knew everyone' and this had a moderating influence on the alcohol-related behaviours of others, particularly under-age drinkers.

Several of the older women interviewed took responsibility for the management of drinking within a club, offering food, asking for proof of age, confiscating car keys or calling a taxi for those drinkers who were obviously inebriated.

> 'Cos I know everyone, I can keep an eye on things. If anyone's being a tool [an idiot], I'll try and have a word with them. Tell 'em to have a softie or some food (Jackie, 65, North Tigers supporter).

> When I'm on the bar, it's easy to see people who've had too much. We're on quite a busy road and there are often breathos [police random breath testing units], so we spread the word about that and call a cab if we need to (Erica, 56, Western Bullets supporter).

This focus on safety and minimising consequences was particularly the case where under-age drinkers were involved. One mother of several junior players notes that:

> I'm often on the door [at club functions], and I run a pretty tight ship. Most of these kids are my son's age, so I know who's old enough to drink. Otherwise,

> you have to show ID, and you get a stamp to get in (Anne, 44, Southern Stars, supporter).

Following on from this, one woman reflected on the broader social networks that were often shared by members of the club, and the way in which these then determined and reflected their own attitude to drinking by minors in a sporting setting:

> Yeah, our kids all went to school together. We've had dinner at their place. They've come to ours. They're pretty relaxed about their kids drinking. I mean they don't want to see them blotto, but if they're at the club, they're happy for their kids to have a couple of beers with them as well. I guess we're pretty responsible about it (Jackie, 65, North Tigers supporter).

The qualitative data indicated that while the women interviewed were happy to refuse or regulate service to minors or to implement strategies such as calling a taxi or suggesting that someone 'slows down a bit', on occasions when male drinkers were excessively boisterous or intimidating, the women drew on the services of male bouncers and security guards when present at a club, or their own husbands or male partners to evict an inebriated drinker.

> If a bloke's getting a bit loud, I might have a word with one of the fellas on the door, and he'll see if he can get him to settle down (Candice, 27, North Tigers supporter).

> It's only happened once, but there was one bloke who was a bit scary. Steve [husband] tried to talk to him, but we ended up calling the cops. It was pretty full on (Louise, 45, Southern Stars supporter).

As such accounts suggest, the football club provided a place where couples and families could come together to socialise and the women were central in organising and managing many of the activities which inevitably involved the service and consumption of alcohol. These 'few good women' (Kelly, et al., 2011) could be characterised as providing a 'civilizing influence' that 'moderated the excesses of male space and made it more attractive for families to encourage their kids to participate' (Kelly, et al., 2011: 481.)

Enforcing morality

While women played an important role in managing the service and consumption of alcohol, this often extended to managing the *moral* dimensions of drinking, particularly that of other women in the club. Although the women interviewed saw excessive drinking as 'just a part of the club' or a 'part of the culture', such acceptance of 'unrestrained, hedonistic and boisterous' (Thurnell-Read, 2011a: 978) behaviour was rarely extended to female drinkers outside of or beyond their own social network:

Well on Saturday like, Jezza's [a player] other half and her friend, when they get together they're bloody shockers … they're just, yeah they just sit in the bar and just drink … that's all I know, but … it's not a good look (Mandy, 32, Eastern Magpies supporter).

Extending this notion of good women as 'moral enforcers', the women interviewed were especially critical of other women who displayed behaviour that was overtly flirtatious or sexual in nature. Discussing a group of women known as 'the Dizzies', the women were particularly disparaging:

We've got this group of girls who sort of hang around, we call them "The Dizzies". Most of them are overweight footy groupies but they tend to drink, well they do, they drink out of control. But I think sometimes they drink to try and impress as well. You can tell what they're out for (Candice, 27, North Tigers supporter).

Here, the women interviewed were critical of drinking displays that were intended to impress or appeal sexually to the men around them. Critically for this narrative, the women interviewed were keen to position groups like the Dizzies as entirely separate from their own drinking activities: 'We just call them The Dizzies because they're, you know, ditzy dizzies. The women, the wives and girlfriends, we don't mix with them. It's a social thing. They drink like a guy. They need to get a hold of themselves' (Deborah, 37, North Tigers supporter).

While the Dizzies' drinking was defined and measured according to men's drinking, and certain limitations were placed around such drinking performances, when reflecting on their *own* drinking, the women interviewed did not subject drinking to excess to the same kind of moral scrutiny, a point to which I will return. Indeed, there was something of a 'double standard discourse' (Lyons and Willott, 2008) in which older women, particularly single older women, were singled out; their behaviours located within broader assumptions about drinking and female respectability (Skeggs, 1997). One of the women interviewed reflected on the fact that 'when it gets late it [the clubrooms] can be a bit like Jurassic Park. It's all older women and I always think "God, go home"'. Another put it far more succinctly: 'They're just embarrassing and look like sluts'.

By contrast, the women interviewed rarely regarded their *own* drinking in these terms. All of the women interviewed perceived occasions of excessive drinking to be 'time out', an opportunity to 'cut loose' or because they had a 'free pass' [a reference to their male partner allowing them a night away from domestic responsibilities]. While such themes of 'cutting lose' or being 'off the leash' are common to accounts of male drinking and are often presented as an archetype of hegemonic masculinity, this is not to suggest that the women involved in this research sought to invert or transgress an established gender order, rather to make the case that the pleasure and enjoyment derived from the sociality of drinking is far from being the preserve of male drinkers alone.

Critically, a discussion of the significant pleasure that women gained from drinking remains something of a discursive oversight in popular narratives of alcohol consumption more broadly, despite it offering a space for relief and respite and a place in which same-sex friendships can be expressed, developed and consolidated (Brown and Gregg, 2012).

Enjoyment and pleasure
Given than many of the women interviewed were involved with a range of volunteer club activities, this imposed certain spatial and temporal limits on their drinking activities. Drinking was often woven into the daily rhythm of attending a game, socialising at the club, then 'kicking on afterwards'. At the game, the women would frequently have a 'chardy' [a chardonnay] and a 'catch up', whilst supporting their husbands, boyfriends or sons who were playing on the day. Here, drinking was a time for women to reflect on life-world issues that were not overly personal or intimate – how the kids are doing at school, the purchase of a new car, an update on a holiday destination and the like. As the day and evening progressed, and drinking moved into the clubrooms, those women who weren't involved with club tasks continued to drink, although this tended to be fairly measured as the women were more often than not, the designated driver.

> Oh, it's a social thing (Mandy, 32, Eastern Magpies supporter).

> Most of my weekends are taken up with the kids' sport, so this is a bit of a chance for me to unwind (Sally, 32, Southern Stars supporter).

> It's a great club. Lots of fun. There's karaoke, and competitions. I really look forward to it … if the boys have won (laughs) (Caitlin, 55, Western Bullets supporter).

> I'm paranoid about breathos on the weekend, so I just have one or two. It's a good laugh, though (Louise, 45, Southern Stars supporter).

As such comments suggest, drinking is clearly a pleasurable activity; a chance to 'unwind' and a place to express the kind of same-sex camaraderie that is commonplace in accounts of male drinking in sport. Such preliminary narratives, however, start to suggest that women's drinking – in this particular sporting context – is subject to a pressure on pleasure; drinking is not as unequivocally 'off the leash' as it more commonly depicted in accounts of men's sport-related drinking where 'competition in the quantity and pace of alcohol consumption' (Peralta, 2007) are central to the 'doing of masculinity through drinking' (Thurnell-Read, 2013: 2). The 'doing' of drinking, in this case, undoubtedly has a performative dimension to it, yet pleasure is not bound to the displays of bodily excess and restraint that we see in accounts of male drinking (Gough and Edwards, 1998; Campbell, 2000; Palmer, 2009; De Visser and McDonnell, 2012).

From Gaps and Silences to New Opportunities

As described here, the preliminary findings of women's understandings and experiences of sport-related drinking offers an account of women's drinking in a particular sporting context – as followers of Australian Rules football in one major Australian city. It does not lay claim to broader generalisations about the relationship between alcohol, sport and female identity, but it does highlight the glaring gap in the literature on gendered discourses about women, sport and alcohol. To return to one of the key themes from the previous chapter, a discussion of drinking pleasures is missing. As Lindsay notes 'drinking alcohol is inherently a social practice strongly associated with pleasure and celebration' (2009: 371), yet the absence of discussion of women suggests that pleasure and celebration, at least in the context of sport-related drinking, are wholly masculine preserves. The qualitative data presented here, however, suggests this is not always the case.

Moreover, the data presented runs counter to the dominant discourse that women drinking, particularly in public, are 'problem women'. The women interviewed here were mothers, wives, and/or club volunteers, several had professional occupations – teachers, lawyers, even an academic – others were students. While the relative homogeneity of the women lays open the possibility for further research with a more diverse range of women with different relationships to alcohol, it is important to note here that all were far from and in no way identified with the caricature of the female binge drinker where a common narrative device is that women behave as 'ladettes' when drunk in public, transgressing normative and dominant forms of femininity by participating in behaviour traditionally defined as male (Day, et al., 2004; Jackson and Tinkler, 2007). In other words, there is a need to move beyond the literature and taken-for-granted orthodoxies so as to not re-inscribe some of the double standards and assumptions about women's drinking.

As I suggested in the previous chapter, the theoretical framing of 'hegemonic drinking' rather than hegemonic masculinity may provide an alternative conceptual lens for rethinking drinking and for (re)framing female drinking in sport. As I have argued in this chapter, dominant, powerful practices and drinking tropes cut across gender, and sport-related drinking is not necessarily about enacting or expressing a particular form of masculinity or transgressing a particular for of femininity. Instead, the preliminary data presented here is a tentative move towards advancing alternative theoretical frameworks for understanding and explaining sport-related drinking. It is tentative, as we know so very little about female drinking in sport, other than perhaps our own anecdotal or personal experiences of sport and, as critical scholars, we need to do more than extrapolate theory from anecdote. Rigorous research is needed. As I have argued elsewhere:

> without substantive empirical research into the presence and meaning of drinking behaviours among women in a sporting context, we run the risk of perpetuating various exclusions of women from key sociological debates and

agendas about sport, identity and the place of alcohol in women's perceptions
and understandings of the two (Palmer, 2011: 172).

It is tentative also as there are two aspects to women and sport-related drinking
that have not been considered here. While some of the women interviewed alluded
to continuing drinking at pubs and nightclubs after the football club and/or as part
of a 'girls night out', an analysis of these activities is beyond the scope of the
current chapter. The focus here is on women's experiences and articulations of
drinking in this particular sporting context, rather than drinking that spills over
into other settings and spaces. Following this, the chapter has not considered how
others may perceive the drinking of female fans on a night out or in situations
where men and women drank together. Women also drank alongside men at
Grand Final celebrations and commiserations and the traditional end-of-season
'Mad Monday' celebrations, and further research on men's perceptions of this
is undoubtedly needed. As Room notes, there is a need to look at 'social and
interactional elements, where gendered roles and often gendered interactions
come into play' (1996: 227), and a consideration of women's drinking 'in the
round' is an important avenue for future research.

Manland: The Politics of Gender

A key space where gendered roles and often gendered interactions 'came into
play' was in terms of my experiences as a female researcher of doing research in
a predominantly male environment and the challenges that went with negotiating
some of the more challenging behaviours by some of the men encountered in
some of the research sites that inform this book. As was the case for Sampson
and Thomas (2003) who conducted their fieldwork aboard a merchant cargo ship
staffed predominantly by men, much of my fieldwork has been conducted in sites
where women were largely absent. Colleagues jokingly dubbed one field site
'Man Land', which somewhat trivialised the discrete politics of gender that I was
constantly having to negotiate in this particular research setting.

Being in, at times, an aggressively masculine environment was highly
confronting. As I document elsewhere (Palmer and Thompson, 2007), being
around football fans while they sang drunken, sexist, racist and homophobic
songs and referred to other women in highly derogatory ways was, at times,
very difficult. My known and overt status as a researcher (discussed further in
Chapters 4 and 9) in no way cushioned me from attitudes and behaviours that I
found personally and profoundly offensive. In such situations, I chose to simply
grin and bear it, a self-conscious strategy that in fact afforded much ethnographic
data about the centrality of such behaviours to the cultural practices of particular
groups of football fans. As Warren notes 'there is a trade off between accepting
sexism on the one hand and the acquisition of knowledge on the other' (1986: 36).

Nonetheless, my own field notes capture the frustrations I felt at having to tolerate such behaviours. Having spent the afternoon with 'the Grog Squad', described elsewhere in the book, during which time two young women in attendance at a football match were continually referred to as 'the Blow Job Girls', purportedly for their willingness to provide sexual favours to some of the players, my fieldnotes from that day included the following entry:

> Spent the afternoon with the Groggies. The familiar (sexist) business as usual was taken to a new level with the naming of two young women/fans as the "Blow Job Girls". I'm aware that my lips thin as I hear this sort of thing, yet I say nothing in the name of "good ethnography". Which it is, but it's hard to reconcile this with my personal politics (field notes, 19 March 2005; Palmer and Thompson, 2007: 203).

As such accounts suggest, aggressively male environments are without question difficult spaces for women to undertake research in, and strategies for managing one's self in the field (such as debriefing or working in pairs) are advised. It is also clear from my field notes that what is observed in the field is filtered by the feelings or beliefs held by the researcher towards the group or individuals concerned. Ethnographies are not dispassionate accounts, and it is sometimes 'difficult to separate fieldwork from our own sense of self' (Coffey, 1999: 68). To present this otherwise would misrepresent both the strength, and the weakness, of the ethnographic method as it relates in this case to research with drinking communities or subcultures.

My response to confronting offensive behaviour is by no means unique. Many accounts of women researching men report a similar lowering of one's own personal or ethical bottom line (Gurney, 1991; Sampson and Thomas, 2003). Gurney, for example, (1985: 45) recalls herself 'turning a blind eye' to comments and innuendo in the field that she would not tolerate in her day-to-day life, while Stanko reports that throughout her research into various aspects of the criminal justice system she was 'continuously reminded of her gender with cat calls and sexualised comments' (1998: 36). As such accounts make clear, women researching men may find their integrity as women, as well as researchers, undermined or called into question, yet as Sampson and Thomas point out, 'failing to challenge such sexist behaviours is not a betrayal of our beliefs, but is [very often] the only practical way to conduct research' (2003: 180).

In light of such observations, what was striking about my fieldwork was the total indifference to me in the field. In other situations, research or otherwise, when a man has used sexist or derogatory language in my company, such utterances are invariably followed by a 'no offence' that was noticeably absent from this particular fieldwork experience. Such gender blindness on the part of my participants, rather than rendering me 'gender-less' (Sampson and Thomas, 2003), in fact *accentuated* my own gendered identity. The total lack of acknowledgement of anything relating to me as a woman (surrounded by men) made me acutely conscious of my gendered self. My femininity was the elephant in the room. As the only woman, there was an unavoidable gender dynamic that shaped the nature of the research, most potently, the relationship between researcher and participant, precisely in the lack of acknowledgement of my presence as a woman.

Conclusion

As outlined previously, the central concern of the book is to 'rethink drinking'; that is, to extend the theoretical and conceptual base of studies of sport-related drinking into new empirical territory. An analysis of women's attitudes towards and their experiences of their own and others drinking is more nuanced than previous theoretical paradigms have done justice to, and falling back on constructions of the gender order in studies of sport, or drinking, simply underscores the omissions and oversights in the scholarship. This is not to suggest we erase gender from the discourse, but to rely on assumptions about male drinking as normal obscures the ways in which women 'do drinking' and the contributions this may make to studies of sports-related drinking and the sociality of alcohol consumption more broadly.

Following Butler's (2004) formulation of 'undoing gender', Markula (2009) has called for new ways of theorisng gender that do not necessarily work to erase the sexes but that avoid conceptualising gender in dichotomous ways. In much the same way that Martin writes of rugby being a 'sexually indifferent environment' where the feminine is absent because both genders are defined on male terms (Martin, 2012: 183), sport-related drinking has similarly been defined in male terms; as conforming to or as resisting assumptions of normative male behaviours.

This, of course, raises, a theoretical issue that is not easily resolved; how do we, can we or do we need to go *beyond* gender in order to challenge gendered understandings of behaviour typically associated with gender? While it has not been my intention to answer that question here, it has been to argue for the advancement of alternative analytical frameworks such as 'hegemonic drinking' or 'calculated hedonism' for understanding the relationships between women, sport and alcohol.

Inasmuch as it has been argued that there is a plurality to masculinities, in sport and elsewhere, there is equally a complexity to drinking (and femininities). As a social practice, drinking is not done, experienced or understood universally. There are different degrees of engagement, and one's relationship to alcohol and sport, for both men and women, intersects with ethnicity, religion, sexuality, and social-economic position, among others. Nonetheless, women's experiences of sport-related drinking has eluded sociological scrutiny, and this chapter has provided a point of departure for a burgeoning research agenda in studies of sport and alcohol.

Chapter 4
Non-drinking, Dry Events and Alternative Forms of Sport

This chapter focuses on:
- non-drinking in environments where strong normative codes of determined drunkenness prevail;
- drinking in alternative forms of sport such as 'lifestyle' sports;
- the implications for hosting and staging sporting mega-events in countries where the consumption of alcohol is prohibited for cultural and/or religious reasons.

Introduction

As I mentioned in the Preface, much of the book is intended as a riposte to the kind of responses I typically receive when I mention my research interests. Before I can declare that my abiding interest is the social contexts of sport-related drinking – the who, how and why of drinking – replies tend to be versions of the following: 'Oh, like hooligans?'; 'Yes, it's terrible. All those guys getting legless and thinking they own the world'; 'Football's the worst, isn't it? Poor old George Best' or 'What do you want to know? Everyone knows they screw around on a night out'. Such responses certainly speak to popular stereotypes and assumptions of sport-related drinking and, to be clear, I am not denying that violence, the exploitation of women or alcohol-related injuries and fatalities exist in particular sporting contexts; there is a rich scholarly tradition that has addressed these, and related issues, and much of this literature has been discussed elsewhere in the book and beyond.

What comments such as 'all those guys getting legless and thinking they own the world' or 'Football's the worst, isn't it?' do, however, is highlight the possibilities for analysis *beyond* these popular stereotypes of sport-related drinking. Some of these possibilities and potentialities are explored in this chapter. Building on the previous chapter, and its focus on women's experiences and understandings of sport-related drinking, the focus of this chapter is on the social meanings and implications of three key areas that deal, essentially, with non-drinking in sport. These are: i) non-drinking in environments where strong normative codes of determined drunkenness prevail; ii) drinking in alternative forms of sport such as 'lifestyle' sports and; iii) the implications for hosting and staging sporting mega-events in countries where the consumption of alcohol is prohibited for cultural and/or religious reasons. The chapter draws empirically on research conducted with British Muslim cricketers in the United Kingdom, with Ultimate Frisbee players in New Zealand, with female roller derby players in the United States, and on an analytical forecasting of the 2022 football World Cup in Qatar. In different ways, these three areas all raise some issues and challenges for alcohol, sport and for promotional and commodity culture more broadly.

Non-drinkers in Sport

Relative to the extensive body of literature that has addressed the negative (and arguably positive) consequences or reasons for drinking and heavy drinking in particular in sport – everything from injuries and fatalities, encounters with the legal system, sexual and physical violence to camaraderie, fun, pleasure and friendship – researchers have focused minimal attention on non-drinkers and how they coexist with drinkers in the particular social setting of sport.

Certainly, a number of sporting clubs and governing bodies have adopted policies such as 'no drinking while travelling'; the headline of 'sobriety at Rio' that I opened the book with follows the Australian Olympic team Chef de Mission for the 2016 Olympic Games call for a ban on alcohol in the Olympic Village and on the return flight to Australia. Similarly, in 2012, Liam Reddy, the Sydney FC goalkeeper was sent home from Wellington, and subsequently sacked from the club for drinking on a flight to New Zealand ahead of a major game. As the football director, Gary Cole put it: 'the team has a firm stance against drinking while in camp and Reddy was sent home for a breach of that policy' (quoted in Blake, 2012).

In a broader research context, non-drinking has been examined in terms of abstinence or non-drinking among recovering alcoholics (Lucas, et al., 2010; Powers and Young, 2008; Schuckit and Smith, 2010) and such studies have been largely quantitative in nature. While useful for identifying patterns and prevalence in a broader adult population, what is missing from such studies is the non-drinkers' – in this case abstinent sportsmen and women – accounts of the social context or the 'definitions of the situation' (Thomas, 1937 in Herman-Kinney and Kinney, 2012: 4) in which non-drinking occurs.

While narrative accounts of alcoholism in relation to sport are discussed in Chapters 5 and 7, both as a biographical and a therapeutic device, my focus in this chapter is on those sportsmen and women who elect not to drink, not as a result of a problematic relationship to alcohol, but through agency and choice, manifested either through their religious beliefs or through an 'aesthetic' belief in care of the self (Foucault, 1988). In terms of pursuing this line of argument, context is, as ever, important to consider. The demographic profile of many sports has changed through migration, ethnic diversity, and shifting relationships to religion and faith, which has led to increasing numbers of sportsmen (and women) choosing not to consume alcohol as a marker of their religion.

Religion and the Cultural Politics of Not Drinking

The intersections between sport and religion raise a whole set of concerns that are beyond the scope of this book (see, for example, Parker and Weir, 2012). Moving beyond the popular metaphor of 'sport as religion', or the notion of sport supplanting the traditional values and expressions of religion, my interest here is with the sorts of questions that religion may pose for negotiating and maintaining particular kinds of relationships – to teammates, to friends and families, and to supporters, among others – in an environment where 'determined drunkenness' (Measham, 2004a) or 'hegemonic drinking' (Palmer, 2013a) occupy places of social and symbolic pre-eminence.

To date, where issues of religion, non-drinking and sport have emerged, they have typically been in terms of elite or professional sportsmen and women. Players such as: Bachar Houli or Hazem El Mazri, who are high profile Muslims in Australian Rules football and Rugby League respectively; Torah Bright, the winner of the women's snowboarding half-pipe at the 2010 Vancouver Games, also a devout follower of the Church of Jesus Christ of the Latter Day Saints (the Mormons); or Tim Tebow, the NFL player noted for displaying Biblical verse on his eye black [the black grease painted under players' eyes to reduce sun glare], for kneeling and praying during games, and for featuring in a pro-life television commercial that aired prior to the 2010 Super Bowl, are among the elite athletes for whom not drinking alcohol is part of their visibly religious presentation of self.

An excerpt from a leading British newspaper provides a brief illustration here. Writing about Torah Bright in the lead up to the 2014 Sochi Winter Olympics, the article describes her as follows:

> Torah Bright: Sochi poster girl or rebellious outsider? Torah Bright, Australian Snowboarder. She was raised a Mormon and says: "I don't drink, smoke, drink tea or coffee, or have sex before marriage" which you can imagine, is not the way most snowboarders live their lives (*Guardian*, 2014).

Empirically, several researchers have examined the experience of Muslim athletes in sport and their relationship to alcohol, although again, the focus has tended to be on the professional or high performance end of sport. Here the work of British academic Dan Burdsey is particularly instructive. Burdsey (2004; 2010; 2011; Burdsey and Randhawa, 2012) has written extensively on the experiences of British Asians in football and cricket, where an exploration and critique of the cultural politics of identity, race and exclusion is at the heart of much of his work. Of interest here is Burdsey's (2010) research on the experiences of British Muslims in first-class cricket, particularly the ways in which the role and significance of Islam in their sporting lives shapes their participation in sport, their relationships to alcohol, and the ways in which this intersects with their experiences of participation in or belonging to a sporting team. In particular, it is the degree to which dominant subcultural and off-field aspects of professional cricket – such as drinking alcohol – are perceived to run counter to observing the obligations of Islam that is of interest here, more specifically, the ways in which interactions between Muslim and non-Muslim cricketers around alcohol consumption highlight some of the politics of exclusion that can accompany sport-related drinking.

Burdsey, for example, notes the 'pejorative discourses and marginalizing practices' (2010: 316) that have surrounded English cricket tours of Pakistan. As Burdsey writes: 'the story often went … being in a Muslim country, the players faced the "unbearable" absence of alcohol' (2010: 316). Reflecting on practice as well as discourse, Burdsey's work recounts 'certain situations and procedures intrinsic to the game of cricket that do not take account of the identities and practices of Muslim players … [such as] … team-mates and club member's frequent consumption of alcohol which, along with other intoxicants, is prohibited (*haram*) in the Qur'an' (2010: 328).

Writing about a county cricket club in the north of England, Fletcher and Spracklen similarly note the ways in which drinking acts as a practice of exclusion among British Pakistani Muslim cricketers, noting that 'ritualized drinking is not and cannot, be enjoyed by all. British Muslims (the majority of whom are of South Asian descent) for instance, are restricted from drinking alcohol due to the demands of Islam' (2013: 1). Drawing on ethnographic research conducted with white British and British Pakistani Muslim cricketers to locate the significance of drinking alcohol in both the inclusion and exclusion of British Pakistani Muslims, Fletcher and Spracklen demonstrate that, in 'negotiating their inclusion, British Pakistani Muslims have to accommodate, negotiate and challenge various forms of inequality and discrimination in their leisure lives' (2013: 1).

While both these pieces of research were conducted in the United Kingdom as (among other things) a window onto the politics and practices of exclusion that can surround non-drinking in sport, they also highlight a gap – both conceptually and geographically – in the wider body of literature. I made the point in Chapter 1 that sport-related drinking (and determined drunkenness more broadly) does seem to be something of a Western problem, so it is here that the work of Yu and Bairner (2012) offers a useful counterpoint, particularly around the kinds of intersections between drinking, religion and exclusion that Burdsey's and Fletcher and Spracklen's work engages with.

Yu and Bairner (2012), in their examination of Confucianism and ethnic stereotyping of Indigenous baseball players in Taiwan, note the ways in which the behaviours of the players 'do little to offset public perceptions about the aborigines as "associated with excessive drinking, singing, joyousness, outgoing personalities and low academic achievement"' (2012: 695). As is the case with other accounts of sport-related drinking, such perceptions are fuelled by the kind of gendered (and in this case racialised) infamy to which I have referred elsewhere – brawling, assaults and encounters with the criminal justice system, among others – in which players become involved.

Of central importance, both Burdsey and Yu and Bairner's work underscores the ways in which drinking – either not doing it or doing too much of it – provides a key lens on race-based exclusionary practices more broadly. Burdsey (2010: 330), for example, notes the ways in which the absence of the behaviour (i.e. not drinking) can spark an interest in and questioning of practices by 'the Other' (why don't you drink?), while displays of drinking by Indigenous baseball players perpetuates particular assumptions that serve to further exclude from sporting interactions and practices those already most marginalised in Taiwanese society (Yu and Bairner, 2012).

Bringing together some of the themes of this chapter with those of the previous chapter, there has also been a growing scholarly interest in Muslim women and sport, which has brought issues of sports participation and religion into sharp relief (Ahmad, 2011; Abdul Razak, Omar-Fauzee and Abd-Latif, 2010; Hargreaves, 2007; Jawad, Al-Sinani and Benn, 2011). While, to date, engaging Muslim women in a dialogue about sport and alcohol has not formed part of this broader inquiry into issues of the body, emancipation, concealment, patriarchy, social inclusion and migration, it does lay open the potential for research into the (perhaps contradictory) place of alcohol in the sporting lives of Muslim women as players or spectators. Once again, the absence of research and scholarship on women and sport-related drinking is highlighted, this time in terms of its absence. As is the case with Burdsey's (2010) research with male Muslim cricketers, questions of inclusion, exclusion and the cultural politics of identity are, in many ways, at the heart of these debates here.

Along with those sportsmen and women for whom non-drinking is foregrounded by religion (in most cases by following the doctrines of Islam), there is also a body of athletes who elect not to drink through personal choice, and these men and women also present fruitful topics for sociological inquiry for what their behaviours might say about athletic austerity, performance and care of the self.

Care of the Self

It is here that I return to the ideas of Michel Foucault introduced in Chapter 2, particularly the notion of 'care of the self'. As discussed briefly then, Foucault's concept of 'care of the self' (Foucault, 1988) was first developed in *Technologies of Self*. There, he was interested in the relationship between structures of domination and the self. Foucault defined technologies of the self as those:

> which permit individuals to effect by their own means or with the help of others
> a certain number of operations on their own bodies and souls, thoughts, conduct,
> and way of being, so as to transform themselves in order to attain a certain state
> of happiness, purity, wisdom, perfection, or immortality (Foucault, 1988: 18).

In terms of how Foucault's ideas have been applied to analyses of sport, care for the self has become glossed somewhat with 'self-care', in which self-care refers to those actions and attitudes which may contribute to the maintenance of wellbeing and personal health, such as diet and exercise. Foucault's ideas have been used extensively in feminist sport scholarship (see Markula, 2003; 2004). Cressida Heyes (2006), for example, in her article 'Foucault Goes to Weight Watchers' considers how self-care practices are built into members' experiences of attending diet and weight-loss centres, in that they provide 'not only a context within which to achieve a culturally desired body but also a sense of self-development, mastery, expertise, and skill that dieting can offer' (2006: 137).

So how then, might these ideas about care for the self or self-care practices be applied to our understandings of non-drinking in the context of sport? Markula's (2003; 2004) articulation of care of the self as necessarily involving a degree of critical awareness is a useful starting point here, for it underpins an awareness by an athlete of what their body is doing and what the athlete is doing to his or her body. Such observations certainly echo with much of the discourse around individual sports such as cycling (Palmer, 1996) or triathlon (Granskog, 1992; Atkinson, 2008). My earlier work on professional cycling, for example, noted the considerable investment in body care that goes into becoming a professional cyclist. As I note elsewhere:

> Issues of diet, sleep or sex are important for framing the cultural aesthetic of cycling. Indeed, there is an enormous range of opinions about effective methods of weight reduction, amongst other things, that testify to the role that these factors play in producing a body type characteristic of the competitive cyclist (Palmer, 1996: 216).

Similarly, Atkinson, writing about triathlon, notes that 'the hyper-health and body orientations that consciously middle-class athletes develop penetrate their everyday assessments of others' eating, exercise, work or relationship habits' (2008: 173). In both cycling and triathlon, care of the self means a critical awareness as to what an athlete is doing to their body and, among elite cyclists or triathletes, the consumption of alcohol, especially anything resembling determined drunkenness, is rarely part of the culture. If anything, *non*-drinking has a certain symbolic capital to it. Abstinence marks a degree of austerity that is necessary to perform well and as such it becomes culturally sanctioned in these sporting communities.

But, what about non-drinkers in team sporting codes and environments where strong normative drinking *do* prevail? How does a non-drinker maintain distinction and symbolic capital (Bourdieu, 1989) given the potential for shared drinking to operate as a form of bonding social capital (Palmer and Thompson, 2007)? Certainly, there are accounts of club enforced periods of non-drinking, or athletes electing not to drink to achieve a competitive edge over their rivals or, indeed, their team mates when competing for squad selection. The start of the 2012 Australian Rules football season, for example, was promoted as 'no booze for Bombers' [the nickname for the Essendon football club] following the announcement that the club would adopt a programme of austerity and restraint:

> From now on I'd imagine 100 per cent of the group will not have a drink. If
> you look at our group there's 39 or 40 players all ready to go, pushing for spots.
> It doesn't take much to find yourself not inside the team. Guys are becoming
> stricter on themselves, more professional. Its what you have to do nowadays.
> Guys respect the footy jumper and they're not going to waste the time they have
> in the jumper by going and doing stupid stuff (Blake, 2012: 17).

But what of those sportsmen and women who consciously elect not to drink
as part of a broader life choice that is not determined by religion but simply a
personal decision? Inasmuch as their choice goes against the grain of normative
expectations of team sport, it raises several questions for how non-drinkers in
these sports negotiate and maintain their identity and relationships to others, given
the centrality of drinking to a range of sports initiations and forms of socialisation
(Clayton, 2012). What, if any, difficulties does it present in different kinds of
sporting (and drinking) contexts? Does this depend on the reason for not drinking;
say, pregnancy or medication, being concerned about maximising sporting
performance, perhaps having struggled with alcohol or other kinds of addictions,
or simply the exercise of a personal choice not to drink?

Drawing on figurational sociology, Atkinson offers a preliminary way of
framing these kinds of questions:

> From a figurational perspective, their subcultural like-mindedness not only
> reflects their collective constructions of the need for meaningful community
> affiliations in/through sport, but also long-term historical trends in Western
> societies that encourage cultural associations between self-restraint, emotional
> control and social distinction, in other terms, "civilised" modes of behaviour
> (2008: 171).

In contrast with the image of reckless and irresponsible drinking behaviours
among sportsmen, such ideas of control and restraint underscore a 'care for the
self' that is underpinned by a Weberian work ethic.

Towards an Analytical Framework for Non-drinkers

The issue of non-drinkers in sport opens up the potential to extend two typologies
that may provide useful analytical frameworks for understanding non-drinkers in
sport. First is the work done by Herman-Kinney and Kinney (2012) on the ways
in which non-drinking college students in the United States formulate, maintain
and transform their personal and social identities. Applying the framework of
'dry' students on a 'wet' campus, Herman-Kinney and Kinney explore the social
experiences of non-drinkers from their own perspectives, examining, in particular,
what it's like to live in an 'environment where drinking is the norm, their moral
experience of stigma and the strategies they employed to develop and maintain
positive experiences identities' (2012: 4).

Alongside this, I, along with colleagues, developed the formulation of 'drinkers, non-drinkers and deferrer' in our work on the culture of alcohol in Australian Rules football among fans of the code (Thompson, Palmer and Raven, 2011). Unsurprisingly, 'drinkers' were those fans that drank, often heavily, while at the football. 'Non-drinkers' abstained from drinking while at the football and in other spheres of their life. 'Deferrers', however, were those who drank little or nothing while at the football, or only drank after the final siren. For deferrers, attending the football 'delayed, discouraged or reduced alcohol consumption, even encouraging abstinence in some cases' (Thompson, et al., 2011: 399). These findings both contrast and challenge previous research that has unequivocally associated (Australian) football with drinking, and, in their presentation of counter-stereotypic ways in which fans engage with alcohol (or not), the authors 'challenge the assumptive worlds in which popular commentary on football and drinking typically operate' (Thompson, et al., 2011: 388).

While both typologies have much analytical utility, and can be usefully extended into other areas where there are entrenched stereotypes at work, there is a risk that such ways of categorising things may prove too blunt, glossing the complexities of the behaviours that sit within the categories of 'wet' and 'dry', or 'drinker', 'non-drinker' or 'deferrer'. Of concern here, sportsmen and women may not always and exclusively be dry (or wet), and may slip in and out of such categories. It is here that more can be done on interrogating the intersections of religion and ethnicity as well as personal choice and agency so as to develop more fine-grained and nuanced understandings of the personal and social identities of non-drinkers in sport.

Drinking and Alternative/Lifestyle Sports

While a section on drinking among participants of alternative or lifestyle sports may seem an odd inclusion in a chapter on non-drinking and sport, it follows as it fits with one of the concerns of the book to pursue counter-intuitive examples and case studies of the sport-alcohol nexus. Ultimate Frisbee and roller derby, I'd hazard a guess, are not among the sports that immediately jump to mind when one thinks about sport-related drinking. In other words, an interest in what I'm calling 'non-normative' forms of drinking, in this case, drinking in sports that go against the grain of some of the popular orthodoxies of sport, and sport-related drinking provides the focus of this particular section.

Before developing the empirical analysis, some preliminary notes on alternative or lifestyle sports are needed to establish the context.

Briefly then, lifestyle sports emerged in the 1960s and have experienced 'unprecedented growth both in their participation and in their increased visibility across public and private space' (Wheaton, 2013: 2). Variously referred to as 'lifestyle', 'action' and 'extreme' sports, the category of activities subsumed includes skateboarding, *parkour*, windsurfing, snowboarding, Ultimate Frisbee, roller derby, kite surfing, canyoning, B.A.S.E jumping and climbing, among others. While encompassing a disparate range of practitioners and geographical sites, scholars such as Stranger (2011) or Wheaton (2003; 2009; 2013) point to the 'outdoor, non-association based and itinerant nature' of these activities (Wheaton, 2013: 4). Moreover, lifestyle sports are seen to represent neoliberal ideologies of flexibility, DIY subjectivity and possibility for all, where the values of individualism, risk-taking, the pursuit of human potential and engaging with one's environment are seen to be common to lifestyle sports (Atkinson, 2009; Wheaton, 2013). In the context of sport-related drinking, notions of individualism, the possibility for all, anti-rules and competitiveness become particularly salient features of this particular sports-scape. The two case studies that follow are emblematic of these alternative or lifestyle sports that are seen to be countercultural in nature; running, in many ways, against, the grain of traditional notions of team sports.

Ultimate Frisbee

As others have noted, Ultimate Frisbee (or 'Ultimate') is an invasion-style team sport played with a flying disc (Crocket, 2013; Griggs, 2011; Thornton, 2004). Key factors which distinguish Ultimate as a lifestyle sport include its origin within the counterculture movement of the 1960s, its code of fair play – Spirit of the Game – being explicitly written into the rules of the game, and, relatedly, players officiating their own games.

Like many other lifestyle sports, Ultimate Frisbee is a 'subculture which values high levels of commitment' (Crocket, 2013: 324). A significant marker of commitment amongst Ultimate players is regular attendance at social and competitive weekend-long tournaments where almost every tournament includes both men and women as active participants. Attending tournaments involves playing multiple games (often seven games per weekend) and a range of associated activities, such as watching other teams play, sharing travel, accommodation and food, and partying.

The socialising between teams, coupled with the values of fair play and self-officiating make Ultimate Frisbee in many ways, something of an 'anti-sport'. Inasmuch as the mixed competition make Ultimate 'an interesting case in which to examine the (re)construction of masculinities' (Crocket, 2013: 319), it similarly offers an interesting case through which to examine the (re)construction of drinking in the context of new forms of sport and leisure. While heavy drinking may well be well critiqued as unhealthy, it is equally implicated in the production of alternative, and potentially less problematic, sporting subjectivities. As I've suggested already, drinking – even heavy drinking – in other words is not always a 'problem', but in some cases, it is both normal and normative in some of our research settings where it provides a rich source of pleasure, enjoyment and sociality.

Hamish Crocket's research on Ultimate in New Zealand suggests that tournament parties, and their associated drinking, form an important part of what it means to be an Ultimate player. As he notes:

Levels of consumption at tournament parties varied significantly, depending on the kind of tournament: thus drinking was timed to the particular event. Parties held during competitive tournaments tended to involve far less determined drunkenness than parties at social tournaments. Typically, heavy drinking at parties revolved around games, such as boat races, three-pint challenges (the amount of beer an upside down Frisbee can hold), and forfeit-based games. Because social tournaments place less emphasis on achieving peak performance, hung over players are not seen as letting their teams down. Instead, I suggest they are seen as having exercised a pleasure-maximising strategy (2014: 10).

To return to the notion of calculated hedonism introduced in Chapter 2, the concept can inform much of the lifestyle surrounding Ultimate Frisbee for it helps facilitate a *contextualised* understanding of heavy drinking or determined drunkenness in Ultimate, which suggests some important contrasts, as well as some similarities with the social relations described elsewhere on drinking in other sports (e.g., Muir and Seitz, 2004; Palmer, 2009; Pringle and Hickey, 2010; Waitt and Warren, 2008). Crockett (2014) points to the mixed nature of Ultimate for explaining some of these contrasts. Ultimate parties feature both men and women as active participants and, so while gender within Ultimate can be constructed in problematic ways (Thornton, 2004), tournament parties nevertheless involve 'practices and tropes which cut across gender' (Palmer, 2013b: 5). Moving beyond gender to frame drinking in Ultimate as involving 'a spectrum of possible positive and negative consequences for the user, for their associates and for wider society' (Measham, 2004a: 316).

Flat-track Roller Derby

As Donnelly (2013) notes in her ethnographic research on women's flat track roller derby, the sport is full-contact, played on a large oval-shaped (flat) track by amateur (unpaid) skaters wearing quad roller skates. In addition to roller skates, the skaters – women of all shapes, sizes, and body types – wear helmets, mouth guards, elbow, wrist and knee pads, as they skate in a variety of venues (e.g. roller rinks, hockey arenas, sports halls, auditoriums, convention centres and parking lots). Skaters' jerseys are often printed with their derby names and numbers. During bouts or 'jams' (roller derby games), announcers typically assist the crowd to follow the action, and music plays between and sometimes during jams. Each two-minute jam features five skaters from each team, playing offense and defense at the same time, officiated by up to seven skating referees and numerous non-skating officials. Announcers, officials, and everybody helping to put on an event are volunteers, and the skaters pay membership dues to play. As was the case with Ultimate Frisbee, women's flat track roller derby is by and large a grassroots sport and many leagues are committed to the do-it-yourself, 'by the skaters, for the skaters' ethics. That is, skaters are the primary owners and managers of the leagues for which they skate, and make most of the decisions (about the sport and the business of roller derby).

Donnelly's (2013) research is useful in the context of non-normative forms of drinking for two reasons. First, as a counter-intuitive or unexpected sport in the context of sport-related drinking, Donnelly's (2013) research compels readers to question some of their assumptions and popular orthodoxies more broadly about the relationships between sport and alcohol and the contexts in which drinking takes place. Second, Donnelly (2013) raises the notion of 'hidden ethnography' as a particular methodological challenge that many researchers working in fields where drugs and alcohol are consumed inevitably face.

While Donnelly's research was not a study of drinking per se, she could not avoid the role that alcohol consumption (of both her research participants' and her own) might play in her research. As Donnelly notes:

> Specifically, and although I was not studying a drinking culture (e.g. a culture organized around or for drinking), I quickly realized that drinking – including being in spaces for drinking, such as bars – was an important part of the social interactions of many of the roller derby skaters I studied. As a result, through the research process, it became clear that I needed to address drinking for two main reasons: 1. the consequences it had for the research process (the conduct of the research); and 2. what it revealed about the social world and about the participants I was studying (2013: 468).

It is the first point that Donnelly makes which is important here, namely the consequences that drinking, particularly, acknowledging it in a study ostensibly not about drinking, may have for the wider research process.

Donnelly recognises that she did not fully anticipate the role of alcohol in her research; a result of what Blackman (2007) calls the 'hidden ethnography'. As Blackman writes, 'there is a disciplinary requirement, and an ethical demand, that the storyteller and the narrative should be "clean". This leads to what can be called the "hidden ethnography", empirical data that is not released because it may be considered too controversial' (2007: 700). Blackman explains that activities such as drinking with participants often become part of the hidden ethnography, and describes his own decision not to include experiences of drinking during his research with young homeless and unemployed people 'because I was unsure how drinking with participants would be interpreted in the discipline, yet it had a major impact in establishing rapport' (Blackman, 2007: 702).

Drinking by and with the derby girls became part of Donnelly's own hidden ethnography for two main reasons. First, the derby girls' drinking, and Donnelly's own drinking, at times crossed boundaries, which raised issues for her research where it 'served as a grey area of interaction and activity that was a part of the social world under study' (Donnelly, 2013: 469). That is, while drinking alcohol was not illegal or 'deviant', it was nonetheless done in ways that were not necessarily 'mainstream' or socially acceptable. Second, drinking by and with the derby girls was relegated to Donnelly's hidden ethnography because these behaviours, actions, and activities appeared to be peripheral to the topic or focus of the research. That is, drinking alcohol was not *the* focus of Donnelly's research but, for various reasons, it attracted her attention and/or become an issue in important ways. Donnelly's focus, in other words, was on women's flat track roller derby as a women-only social formation, and not on the drinking or partying of 'derby girls'.

By contrast, my own research on the social meanings of drinking in Australian Rules football was explicitly a study of alcohol consumption, so my ethnography of drinking could in no way be hidden. In my case, it was imperative that I was entirely transparent about my purpose for visiting football matches and spending time in the various contexts and settings where drinking took place. Like other research where gaining and maintaining access depends on good relations with gatekeepers and respondents (Sampson and Thomas, 2003; Belousov, et al., 2007), my research was openly presented as being 'for a book about sport and drinking'. To support such professional claims, I always carried university identification. On the odd occasion when I was asked to verify my credentials as an academic researcher, my identification was viewed with little more than a cursory glance and handed back to me with the inevitable response of 'you've got a cushy number [job] haven't you? Do you get to do this every weekend'?

Drinking on the Job: The Politics and Pragmatics of Fieldwork with Drinking Communities

Being seen to drink alcohol also provided a crucial point of entry into the culture of alcohol in Australian Rules football I was interested in learning more about (see Figure 4.1). It exposed me to many of the practices associated with drinking, such as buying in rounds, drinking with non-drinkers, 'pacing and chasing' and opting out. I noted that drinking outlets were separated according to alcoholic or non-alcoholic beverages and I soon realised why people buying a round or a 'shout' were reluctant to order a non-alcoholic drink as it meant sending the 'shouter' to queue at a separate and often distant outlet. In other words, the consumption of alcohol became fundamental to the research process in terms of the access it granted me and the ways in which it then legitimated my presence in the field. In many ways, being seen to drink was more important in securing my continued access to the field than the more formal negotiation of gatekeepers. As Sampson and Thomas note 'being in a fieldwork setting and gaining initial access to a site is no guarantee of acceptance, much less trust or even popularity. Hard won trust and rapport can be quickly lost in the face of a perceived rejection or "social snub"' (2003: 174).

Such admissions to drinking on the job may invite criticism from those who uphold the view that the task of the researcher is to retain some degree of critical distance and judgement, particularly when in potentially volatile situations such as the highly masculine environment of football where alcohol is consumed. As a female researcher, surely I was inviting trouble? Following Armstrong (1993) who became firm friends with some of the violent, hooligan informants at the centre of his study or Thornton (1995) who shared capsules of MDMA (ecstasy)

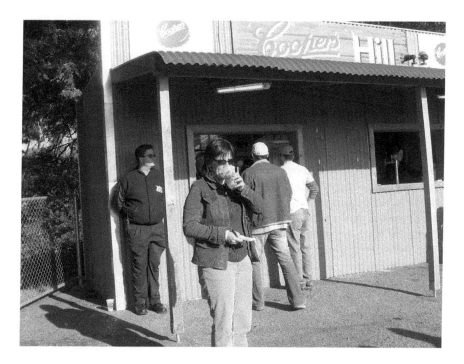

Figure 4.1   Drinking on the job

Source: Photograph author's own.

with her informants in her ethnography of club culture in Britain, I contend that some fieldwork situations necessitate ethnographers engaging in the behaviours he or she is interested in knowing more about, even if this blurs some of the boundaries and roles of researcher and participant (Sherif, 2001). My visible alcohol consumption was a deliberate research strategy to facilitate my fieldwork. It offset the perception that I was taking the moral high ground and it provided direct and intimate access to the very attitudes, behaviours and practices I had been commissioned to document and detail. In this respect, it would have been less appropriate to abstain than to indulge.

Alcohol and 'Dry' Mega-events

One of the more interesting – and rapid – developments in considering the sport-alcohol nexus has been the need to consider the implications of alcohol sponsorship and consumption when sporting mega-events are held in countries and regions where the sale and/or consumption of alcohol is forbidden. This section then, looks at some of the implications of hosting the 2022 FIFA World Cup in Qatar; an

Islamic country where the 'use of alcohol is especially troubling for Muslims, who may be deeply offended if they are in the vicinity of alcohol' (Dun, 2014: 186). I offer first however, some more general observations on the nature of the sporting mega-event and their rapid expansion into non-Western countries.

The Sporting Mega-event

Mega-events are key events for sport and for social scientists as particular sites or subjects of analysis. These 'large-scale cultural events, which have a dramatic character, mass popular appeal and international significance' (Roche, 2000: 1), be they rock concerts, the inaugurations of political leaders, World Expos or, in this case, sporting events like the Olympic Games or football's World Cup, are quintessential phenomena of global modernity; 'intrinsically complex processes, which combine the interests of political and economic elites and professionals from the increasingly supranational cultural industries' (Roche, 2003: 99).

Moreover, the social and economic impacts of sporting mega-events in terms of urban regeneration, tourism benefits or legacy outcomes for the cities and countries who host them have all been recognised by governments, non-governmental organisations and 'cosmocrats' alike. Indeed, hosting major sports events has, for a number of countries, been an important element in tourism promotion (Sydney 2000 Olympic Games, South Africa's 2010 FIFA World Cup, Rio 2016 Olympic Games) and in urban and social regeneration (Barcelona 1992 Olympic Games, 2010 Commonwealth Games in Delhi, London 2012 Olympic Games), while 'urban revitalization' has become official policy in the European Union, in individual states and in specific cities (Gratton and Henry, 2001).

The growing global capital that non-Western countries now exercise has seen a number successfully bid for a whole host of sporting events, including football's World Cup, the Olympic Games, Formula One Grand Prix, cricket tournaments and international athletics and cycling competitions. As Curi, Knijnik and Mascarenhas note:

> It has become common for former so-called semi-peripheral developing countries to stage sports tournaments of global significance: the 2008 summer Olympic Games in Beijing, the 2010 Commonwealth Games in New Delhi, the 2014 Winter Olympics in Sochi and the 2014 FIFA World Cup in Brazil and the 2016 Summer Olympics in Rio de Janeiro (2011: 141).

Indeed, a number of countries beyond the traditional economic power triad of North America-Europe-Japan have successfully bid for the right to host sporting mega-events, which has shifted conceptualisations of them (both the country and the mega-event).

Qatar, for example, has carved out a global niche in hosting sporting mega-events in the Gulf States. As Campbell notes 'state investment in technologically and architecturally first-rate facilities has helped qualify Qatar as a global participant' (2010: 49). The International Association of Athletics Federations Championships, the Qatar Moto GP, the 2011 Asian Cup, the Tour of Qatar cycle race and the 2022 FIFA World Cup are just a few of the high profile sporting events to be staged in Qatar. It is the 2022 FIFA World Cup that is of particular interest here in the context of the sport-alcohol nexus. Qatar is an Islamic state where the consumption of alcohol in public is prohibited under Sharia Law on which the Qatari legal system is based.[1]

For many, the absence of alcohol at a major sporting event is viewed as an anathema to attending a major sporting mega-event. As Gee, Jackson and Sam note 'some football fans cannot seem to conceptualize attending matches in which they cannot consume alcohol beverages before, during or after it; it is in an inherent component of their identity as fans and is a key behaviour necessary to enact the role' (2014: 7). Gee's (2013) (auto)ethnographic account of the processes that link the social, political and cultural representations of alcohol sponsorship with the 2011 Rugby World Cup in New Zealand, for example, recounts the Prime Minister of New Zealand, Rt Hon John Key, as 'being among the first to describe Auckland's waterfront Queens Wharf area as "Party Central" during the tournament: 'This will be "party central" – the focus of a mass public opening ceremony and the magnet for fans who can't be at games during the six-week tournament' (Gee, 2013: 924). Further, Gee describes the extent to which aspects of popular culture more broadly are routinely appropriated in ways that promote the wholesale consumption of alcohol during major sporting events, in this case the 2011 Rugby World Cup:

> Supermarkets, for example New World (a nationwide supermarket chain in New Zealand), featured large displays of Heineken cans, bottles and Draught Kegs (a mini keg that gives 20 £ 250 ml serves) with special drink deals. When customers purchased a Heineken product, they received a Heineken Hosting Guide outlining how to celebrate the 2011 RWC in true Heineken style. Topics in this guide include a checklist for the perfect Heineken host, optimal room set-up, RWC party theme options, ideas for snacks, clean-up tips and tricks and being a perfect guest (Gee, 2013: 925).

While the presentation of mega-event sites and cities as being 'party central' spaces is undoubtedly part of the discourse and indeed the experience of spectacles like the Rugby World Cup, this becomes problematic for the implementation of public and health policy and legislation in some of the nations in which mega-

---

1   Intoxicants were forbidden in the Qur'an through several separate verses revealed at different times over a period of years. At first, it was forbidden for Muslims to attend to prayers while intoxicated (4:43). Then a later verse was revealed which said that alcohol contains some good and some evil, but the evil is greater than the good (2:219). This was the next step in turning people away from consumption of it. Finally, 'intoxicants and games of chance' were called 'abominations of Satan's handiwork', intended to turn people away from God and forget about prayer, and Muslims were ordered to abstain (5:90–91)

events are due to take place, or have taken place recently. Brazil, for example, the host nation of the 2014 football World Cup experienced the iron fist of *Fédération Internationale de Football Association* (FIFA – the global governing body for football) who coerced the Brazilian government to change a law that has prohibited the sale of alcohol in Brazilian sports stadiums since 2003 in order to protect the commercial rights of the American beer company Budweiser, one of its World Cup sponsors. According to FIFA General Secretary, Jerome Valcke:

> Alcoholic drinks are part of the FIFA World Cup, so we're going to have them. Excuse me if I sound a bit arrogant but that's something we won't negotiate. The fact that we have the right to sell beer has to be part of the law (BBC News, 2012a).

Moreover, this law change was part of the conditions stipulated by FIFA when Brazil was awarded the 2014 World Cup.[2] In June 2012, the Congress and President of Brazil eventually passed the highly publicised and nicknamed 'Budweiser Bill' (BBC, 2012b). Indeed, this case highlights the power of one global governing sports body to influence amendments to pre-existing nation-state legislation to preserve alcohol sponsorship rights to sports events.

So what then for Qatar? Will we see a similar overturning of laws? Will we see the FIFA exert similar pressures on the Qatari government to protect the commercial rights of corporations like Budweiser? I have argued elsewhere that transnational organisations like the International Olympic Committee or FIFA have 'developed an extra-ordinary capacity for self-authority that is rarely challenged' (Palmer, 2013c: 43) and certainly, the evidence from Brazil suggests that FIFA is a 'powerful organization ... which enjoy[s] wealth, celebrity status and global influence on a scale with few rivals' (Palmer, 2013c: 52). But, looking ahead to the football World Cup in Qatar in 2022, to what extent may – or will – FIFA's self-authority be moderated or challenged by Islamic beliefs and Sharia Law? While Qatar 2022 is still eight years away at the time of writing, what has become known as the Qatari compromise raises some important questions for the global politics of not only sport but the commercial reach of the alcohol industry, and its promotional culture.

The Qatari Compromise

While the consumption of alcohol is not illegal in Qatar, drinking in public or being drunk in a public place – often a very public feature in media coverage of fan's experiences of sporting mega-events – can result in monetary fines, deportation or even prison sentences. Muslims who are caught drinking may be

---

2   The debate over alcohol sales at World Cups is not limited to Qatar or Brail. Russia, which is hosting the 2018 World Cup, prohibits alcohol at stadiums and nearby stores. President Vladimir Putin in January, 2014, promised FIFA president Sepp Blatter that it would reconsider a ban on beer at stadiums during the World Cup.

subject to corporal punishment. With alcohol consumption so tightly regulated during 'normal' life in Qatar, to what extent will calculated hedonism, so much a part of a fan's experience of travelling to and attending events like the World Cup, be curtailed by the broader regulatory processes of Sharia Law? Will FIFA exert similar kinds of pressure on Qatari lawmakers to those placed on the Brazilian government? How will Qatar respond? Such questions are speculative, but early indications suggest something of a compromise has been reached to allow alcohol to be consumed in public during the World Cup in order for FIFA to preserve its alcohol sponsorship rights to sports events and for the sport-alcohol nexus to remain intact for fans travelling to Qatar. Hassan Abdulla al Thawadi, chief executive of the Qatar 2022 World Cup bid has already indicated that specific 'fan-zones' will be created where alcohol can be bought and consumed.[3]

Clearly, broader cultural assumptions and national stereotypes are at play here. Dave Richards, the Chair of the English Premier League has stated that Qatar would have to strike a balance between pleasing European soccer fans who enjoy a pint with the cultural sensitivities of the Gulf nation where drinking alcohol is discouraged.

> In our country and in Germany, we have a culture. We call it, "We would like to go for a pint and that pint is a pint of beer". It is our culture as much as your culture is not drinking. There has to be a happy medium. If you don't do something about it, you are starting to bury your head in the sand a little bit because it needs addressing. You might be better off saying don't come. But a World Cup without England, Germany, the Dutch, Danes and Scandinavians – it's unthinkable (Richards, 2012).

Given the recent actions of FIFA in relation to the 2016 football World Cup in Brazil, the statements made by FIFA officials about the 2022 World Cup in Qatar, suggest that FIFA will, in all likelihood, require that alcohol be available and without restrictions such as fan zones, as well as relaxing the penalties for the public consumption of alcohol and public drunkenness. As Dun notes 'lashing or deporting fans for violating alcohol laws would certainly create a scandal on a magnitude Qatar does not desire and it would be a further blow to their soft power strategy in hosting mega-events' (2014: 197).

Conclusion

This chapter has been concerned with unpacking some of the social meanings and implications of non-drinking and non-normative forms of drinking in sport.

---

3   Similar fan zones that were trialled during the 1996 European Championship in England proved popular with fans who would drink all day and watch the games, unlike Premier League games in England where alcohol is sold at stadiums, but fans cannot drink in view of the field.

Drawing on research conducted with British Muslim cricketers in the United Kingdom, with Ultimate Frisbee players in New Zealand, with roller derby players in the United States, and on an analytical forecasting of the 2022 World Cup in Qatar, these three examples all raise particular issues and questions for alcohol, sport and for promotional culture more broadly. Indeed, the presence of athletes who choose not to drink for religious reasons, when overlaid against a broader discourse of multiculturalism and ethnic diversity, makes a discussion of non-drinking in sport a useful point of entry into debates of inclusion and exclusion, belonging and identity more broadly. Equally, there is clearly a range of reasons for not drinking by both athletes and sports consumers alike, which leave open potential analyses of questions of legitimacy, authenticity, agency, identity, belonging, health and body care and care for the self for further exploration through empirical research.

Similarly, 'non-normative forms' of drinking; that is, drinking in sports that go against the grain of some of the popular orthodoxies of sport, and sport-related drinking (in this case Ultimate Frisbee and women's flat track roller derby) offer some counter-intuitive examples of the sport-alcohol nexus that challenge popular orthodoxies of sport-related drinking. In terms of the global politics and economics of sport, the decision to host the 2022 FIFA World Cup in Qatar, an Islamic state where the consumption of alcohol in public is prohibited under Sharia Law, raises a whole set of questions about promotional culture, religion, 'the Other' and the centrality of sponsorship by alcohol companies to the hosting of major, global sporting mega-events that will unfold over the coming years.

Chapter 5
Biographies of Drinking

This chapter:
- examines narratives of alcohol 'addiction' among professional and elite level athletes;
- analyses four key biographies or autobiographies that recount the story of an athlete's struggle with their addiction to alcohol.

'The only person who would have spent more time on the ice than me was Ben Cousins'

In a speech to players at the launch of the 2012 season for AFL club, the West Coast Eagles, Steven Bradbury – the Australian speed skater who infamously won gold at the 2002 Winter Olympics when the entire field in front of him crashed out – alluded to the drug use of Cousins, a celebrated, former West Coast player. Bradbury's double entendre – a nod to his own sport and to Cousins' battles with methylamphetamine (or 'ice') addiction – went down like a lead balloon. Cousin's suspension in 2009 from the AFL for 'bringing the game into disrepute', his own admission to drug use and addiction and subsequent time spent in drug and alcohol rehabilitation centres, is among the more high profile cases of the problematic use of drugs and alcohol by elite athletes, and his story opens up a dialogue on other sportsmen and women battling drug and alcohol addictions.

As I develop in this chapter, there has been something of a discursive shift in how the drinking and drug-taking behaviour of sportsmen (sportswomen being almost entirely absent) has been received and debated in popular and press accounts. The veneration of sportsmen for heavy drinking is (arguably) declining, tempered now by a discourse that is suggestive of a duty-of-care, restraint, governance and surveillance by sports clubs and officials. At the same time, the development of specialist drug and alcohol treatment centres for sportsmen and women (notably, Tony Adams' Sporting Chance Clinic in the United Kingdom) suggests that drug and alcohol misuse among athletes is emerging as a significant social problem. As others have noted, many sportspeople – professional footballers in particular – suffer from addiction to drugs and alcohol (Dunning and Waddington, 2003; Gogarty and Williamson, 2009; Roderick, 2006), with George Best, Jimmy Greaves, Paul Gascoigne, Tony Adams, Paul McGrath, Paul Merson and Dean Windass being among the more high profile British players who have battled addiction.[1] As I discuss shortly, their difficulties often come to light in tabloid media where they are represented as 'fools' or 'villains' following an off-field misdemeanour (Lines, 2001). These stories of drinking, downfall and redemption are among the central themes explored in the following pages.

With this as background, the concern of this chapter is to examine some of the narratives of alcohol 'addiction' among professional and elite level athletes, particularly their 'fall from grace', their decline, recovery and, in some cases, their death. Sport may have a rich tradition of famous drinkers – Brendan Fervola in Australian Rules football or the American golfer John Daly being added to some of the names above – yet their behaviours, and how the 'story' around these behaviours is recounted and remembered, has not yet been sustained to a systematic, sociologically informed analysis.

Utilising the concept of 'interpretive framing' (Silverman, 2013) this chapter analyses four key biographies or autobiographies that recount the story of an athlete's struggle with addiction to alcohol in particular. The chapter outlines some of the contradictory themes or fault lines that run through narratives of addiction in professional sport. The chapter locates the discussion within broader debates about responsibility, notions of 'addiction', entitlement and scandal that then set the scene for the second half of the book, which shifts its focus to re-dressing the problem of alcohol misuse in sport, particularly some of the culture change and treatment and prevention programmes that the use and misuse of alcohol by professional athletes discussed in this chapter helps to make maximally visible.

Four biographies are discussed, each focussing on a different sport and different sporting identity. These are *Addicted* by former England footballer Tony Adams; *My Life in and Out of the Rough: The Truth Behind All That Bull***** by former US golfer John Daly; *Footballer: My Story* by former captain of the English women's football team, Kelly Smith; and *From the Eye of the Hurricane: My Story*, by former Irish snooker player, Alex Higgins. These texts have been chosen, not because they are in any way representative of the issues, but because they offer sources of data that provide 'deep insights into subjective expressions of experience' (Stewart, et al., 2011: 583), in this case, alcoholism and addiction.

Methodological and Theoretical Context

During the last two decades, personal and autobiographical narrative accounts have become increasingly common in empirical research studies in sport. Used

---

1   George Best was a Northern Irish professional footballer who played for Manchester United. Jimmy Greaves is a former England international footballer. Paul Gascoigne is a former England international footballer. Tony Adams is a former Arsenal and England international footballer who established the Sporting Chance treatment centre in 2000. Paul McGrath is a former Irish international footballer. Paul Merson is a former Arsenal and England international footballer. Dean Windass is a former Hull City footballer.

primarily as an autoethnographic device, researchers situate themselves in their field, most often as a participant in the activity under study (e.g., Allen Collinson and Hockey, 2005; 2007; Jones, 2006; Lyons, 1991; Sparkes, 1996; 1998; 2002; Sugden, 1997; Young, et al., 1994).

At the same time, biographical/autobiographical accounts from sporting identities line the shelves of bookshops, where (auto)biographies have become something of a stock in-trade for high profile athletes. There is no shortage of texts which celebrate the successes of sports stars in a variety of sports and they often they follow a predictable chronological format tracing the athlete's life from childhood through adolescence to adulthood and stardom – and also sometimes to decline. Tulle (2014) draws attention to the passage of time in the making and unmaking of the narratives and biographies that surround the making and unmaking of sports stars. As I will return to, stories of 'place'; that is, accounts of where sportsmen and women grew up and, in some cases, learned to drink, are similarly central to many of the (auto)biographies of the making, unmaking and re-making of addicted sportspeople, footballers in particular.

In most sporting (auto)biographies, the broad narrative unfolds in one of two ways: remembering a remarkable life or recounting a remarkable achievement. Biographies dealing with addiction tend to fall into the category of the former, and the richness of some of these remarkable lives is highlighted shortly. As I will return to, sporting (auto)biographies also bring to life the sociological imagination, enabling us to 'grasp history and biography and the relations between the two in society' (Mills, 1959: 6). Indeed, as Stewart, et al. (2011: 583) suggest, published autobiographies are a potentially rich, but neglected source of data for what they might suggest about wider social relations and struggles.

Biographies as Data Sources

Autobiographies – literally meaning the description of one's own life – are a useful source of data to which various forms of analyses can be applied in order to generate insights into and enhance our understanding of social relationships and activities as experienced by the individuals who live through them (Stewart, et al., 2011: 583). Tulle (2014), for example, in her analysis of the retirement of male athletes from competitive sport, where she examines the biographies of Roger Federer (Jaunin, 2007) and Lance Armstrong's (2004) ghosted autobiography, *Every Second Counts*, draws on these sources to examine larger questions about ageing, the making and unmaking of modern athletic careers and the service of the body to the dehumanising modern apparatus of contemporary sport.

Although immensely rich and rewarding sources of data that can place a sporting star's life in a broader socio-historical context, the use of biographies and autobiographies, like other data sources, is not without its limitations. As Jones notes 'autobiographies are potentially unreliable, in that they are often ghost written and edited, they can be overly sentimental and may fail, therefore to provide an honest account' (2014: 488). Similarly, Leskelä-Kärki (2008) acknowledges that 'the borders of fictional texts and autobiographical accounts are complex and shifting' (2008: 327), calling for a wider understanding of the discursive frames within which analyses sit in order to then subject them to critical scrutiny. Stanley's theorising of the term 'auto/biography' is useful here, because it disturbs the supposed binaries of self and other, fact and fiction, past and present, reality and representation, autobiography and biography, pointing out how these intersect in different narratives to produce counter narratives, resistant readings and various versions of differently but equally valid 'truth' about and by the subject in question (Stanley, 1992).

In this vein, narratives of addiction, and auto/biographical accounts of dependence on alcohol, decline and recovery are almost unavoidably blurry affairs where memories of the past may compromise the honesty of an account in the present. Certainly, misty memories of halcyon days gone by – of an athlete's star rising rather than their falling – also play a part in distorting a linear account of the life of an individual, irrespective of their athletic performance. While acknowledging the limitations of historical memory, my concern here is less with a quest for 'truth' or to validate the reliability of autobiographical accounts and more to explore the potential of auto/biography to locate, conceptually, stories of addiction within an athlete's social and sporting life more broadly.

As suggested already, a key dimension to accounts of alcohol addiction is that of 'place'; that is, stories of the places where people drink, their drinking environments – the pubs, the homes, the public spaces – as well as where they grew up and, in some cases, learned to drink – form key parts of the narrative. While the focus in this chapter is on stories of alcohol and stories of addiction, Chapter 7 adopts a different perspective on telling stories or talking about alcohol and addiction, where it discusses the use of narrative as a therapeutic device in recovery.

Analysing Biographies

Given some of the limitations with the use of (autobiographies) as data sources, in this chapter, I bring together several methodological threads to draw out my analysis. Using Silverman's (2013) notion of 'interpretive framing' in which key themes in the biographical texts are translated into recognisable cultural scripts or narratives, I subject the four key (auto)biographies that I will come to in a moment to this process. Alongside this, I employ the concept of 'media framing', used elsewhere in cultural and media studies to understand the ways in which producers of texts – be they media texts such as films or television programmes or written texts such as those (auto)biographies that interest me here – construct and present particular representations of reality.

Gamson conceptualised the media frame as 'a central organizing idea used for making sense of relevant events', which can provide a basis for exploring how readers may 'understand and remember a problem' (1989: 157) while, similarly, Gitlin defined media frames as 'persistent patterns of cognition, interpretation, and presentation, of selection, emphasis, and exclusion' (1980: 7). In my analysis of the sporting (auto)biographies, this notion of 'framing' and the interpretive assumptions built into it, à la Silverman (2013), provides a methodological framework for guiding the analysis of the four auto/biographies discussed in order to identify the specific properties and themes that give shape and meaning to the narrative.

Specifically, this form of framing analysis employs Altheide's (1996: 23–44) process of 'document analysis' to connect the textual representations that are the focus of the study (the auto/biographies) to broader ideas in discourse and ideology, such as notions of addiction, duty-of-care, restraint, governance and surveillance. Altheide's approach defines the conceptual relationship of discourse, themes, and frames as follows: 'the actual words and direct messages of documents carry the discourse that reflects certain themes, which in turn are held together and given meaning by a broad frame … Frames are a kind of "super theme"' (1996: 31).

This method of document analysis involves developing the context for the sources of documents to be analysed, in this case the sporting and/or social milieu that shaped their lived experience as athletes with developing addictions; examining a small number of the documents – in this case the four auto/biographies – to begin developing themes and categories to guide then the analysis of the data, which involves extensive reading, sorting, and searching through the documents (or auto/biographies), comparing and contrasting extremes and key differences, summarising findings, and then integrating or overlapping the findings with interpretation (Altheide, 1996: 31). This leads to the generation of certain cultural scripts that unfold along particular narrative lines, and in the section that follows, I outline the key texts under discussion before returning to these cultural scripts that emerged from the document analysis, to interrogate them with broader conceptual interpretations drawn from theories of place and illness and recovery, among others.

(Auto)biographies of Addiction

Four (auto)biographies frame the analysis that follows:

1. *My Life In and Out of the Rough: The Truth Behind All That Bull***** is the 'candid memoir' of the 1991 PGA Champion, John Daly. Written with Glen Waggoner, but in the first person of Daly, *My Life* (2006) recounts Daly's struggles with alcohol, gambling and sex addictions. As described in the publisher blurb: it is a 'chart of celebration and self-destruction'.
2. *Eye of the Hurricane: The Alex Higgins Story* (Hennessey, 2000) recounts the life of Alex 'Hurricane' Higgins, the former British snooker player who won the 1972 World Championship. Reading more like the 'tour diary of a rock 'n' roll hell raiser than a professional snooker player', *Eye of the Hurricane* traces Higgins' battles with alcohol and the throat cancer that eventually killed him.

While the key themes – or cultural scripts in Silverman's (2013) terms – to emerge from these two (auto)biographies will be elaborated shortly, the important point here is that both of these sportsmen (and I use sports*men* deliberately) conform to what Whannel (1999) describes as 'maverick sport stars' whose 'athletic mastery is expressed in their ability to display creative genius apparently unhindered by discipline or a traditional work ethic in training' (Tulle, 2014: 3). Maverick sport stars, it has been suggested (Tulle, 2014), capture our imagination because they are unpredictable and vulnerable to downfall, the result of moral and physical decadence in equal measures (Archetti, 2001).

As I elaborate shortly, accounts of maverick sports stars like Daly or Higgins, often focus on their deviant behaviour when drunk, such as driving under the influence, infidelity, violence, and breaking team rules. Daly, for example, is described as the 'unapologetic bad boy of professional golf', while Higgins 'created his own high-octane atmosphere, roaring flames of defiance and generally shoving two fingers up to society'. Behind the 'deviance' or 'vice' narratives, however, are complex stories of suffering and chaos.

By contrast, the third (auto)biography *Addicted* (Adams, 1998) by former English football captain, Tony Adams describes less a 'maverick' sports star and more an athlete battling parallel addictions – to alcohol and to professional football. As the title suggests, *Addicted* offers an insight into what addiction is like; how addiction develops and how it affects lives and careers.

Similarly, the fourth (auto)biography *Footballer: My Story* by former captain of the English women's football team, Kelly Smith (2012), traces her success as a player and her battles with alcohol. Smith's story is one of the few accounts of a female athlete struggling with an addiction to alcohol and it returns us to some of the themes introduced in Chapter 3. As I noted then, 'the broad characterisation [of women's drinking] unfolds in one of two ways: women's lives are worse than men's and therefore they take drugs and use alcohol to make their lives better or, for younger women in particular recreational/celebratory that is bound up in a discourse of risk taking' (Measham, 2003: 22). As I suggest in what follows, accounts such as Smith's bring together these twin discourses of risk and celebration and 'escape' from sadness and uncertainty.

Key Themes and Cultural Scripts

As Jones notes 'there is little or no published research which seeks to better understand what it is like to suffer from alcoholism from the perspective of the player-addict themselves' (2014: 486). From the four (auto)biographies discussed here, several key, intersecting themes emerge: an overarching restitution narrative; and then, within that, the subthemes of: i) fighting against illness; ii) the journey; and iii) the return.

These cultural scripts are similar to those identified by Stewart, et al. (2011) in their analysis of the themes and metaphors they found in 12 autobiographies that they studied of athletes with chronic illness, including cancer, HIV and rheumatoid arthritis. More than simply rhetorical flourishes, metaphors can have a powerful influence on the experience of illness and addiction. Treating addiction (to alcohol) as an illness, similar themes emerge from the auto/biographies under study here.

Restitution Narrative

The 'restitution narrative' was first coined by the health sociologist Arthur Frank (1991). According to Frank, the restitution narrative has the basic storyline: 'Yesterday I was healthy, today I'm sick, but tomorrow I'll be healthy again' (Frank, 1991: 85).

In the case of the (auto)biographies, we see this narrative of the restoration of the self in the story of Tony Adams. Describing his decline and recovery from self-admitted alcoholism, Adams's biography reads:

> Tony Adams is one of the legends of English football. An inspirational captain, he's also amassed more than 50 England caps. But Adams has also had his problems over the years. He was jailed after being convicted of drink driving, left out of England's 1990 World Cup squad; needed 29 stitches after falling down a flight of stairs in a nightclub and finally, in the summer of 1996, admitted he was an alcoholic. This is the story of a winner; a man who has shown the strength of character and mental strength to regain the captaincy of club and country and continues to set new goals in his life (1998: cover notes).

A similar theme of 'bouncing back' shapes the cultural script of Kelly Smith's autobiography. The publisher blurb again is instructive here:

> Kelly Smith is the greatest women's footballer that this country (England) has ever produced. Yet for a shy girl from Watford, it has been a long and difficult journey to the pinnacle of the world game, and one which involved the hardest of challenges. Lonely, thousands of miles from home at college in the United States, a series of career-threatening injuries led to severe depression and a battle with alcoholism. But with her typical fighting spirit, Kelly bounced back to inspire Arsenal to countless trophies and to write her name in the history books as England's record goal scorer (2012).

It is this overarching theme of the 'descent' into alcohol abuse, the admission of the problem and the subsequent challenge to regain their mental and physical health that links these two autobiographies of athletes with very different life stories.

Fighting against illness
Metaphors of war, battle or fight often used to frame self-stories or biographies in a sporting context are also part of the cultural scripts through which admissions of illness, in this case addiction, are articulated. Adams, for example, recalls that

'gradually, I was losing everything and the drink was winning ... I was a footballer, a winner. But I was the winner who had lost when it came to alcohol' (1998: 15), while both Smith and Daly describe drinking as an 'enemy to fight'.

The metaphor of war works, I'd suggest, as it has cultural resonance more broadly (the 'wars' on drugs, terrorism or poverty, for example) and it connotes a seriousness of purpose that offsets the 'powerlessness' of an alcoholic over their illness or addiction. John Daly, for example, writes that:

> if I was still drinking whiskey, I wouldn't be drinking anything right now, I'd be dead. That's the truth and I know it. The first time I came out of rehab, in 1993, I said I was never going to drink again. The second time I came out of rehab, in 1996, I said I would never drink again. Now I just pray I never drink whiskey again, because if I do, I know it'll kill me (2006: 154).

In all of the featured (auto)biographies, alcoholism was an insidious evil that 'snuck up' on them, and against which they then had to fight or battle. Tony Adams, for example, writes that:

> It was dawning on me that I couldn't beat the booze ... . I thought, as I stood here alone at the bar ... I had no choice in the matter, again. Why was that? As yet, though I was getting stirrings that I might be suffering from the illness of alcoholism, I had no real insight into its insidious nature and though I had shown than I could stop for short periods, I had no idea how to stay off the booze permanently. Didn't want to know. Who wants to be an alcoholic? (1998: 13).

Similarly, Smith writes of 'drinking so hard [she] could no longer feel her senses' (2012: 91) and of trying to tell herself '"don't have a drink today Kelly". But I would fail in that quest. I found I needed a drink. That I had to have a drink. I absolutely hated myself for drinking as much as I did but I just couldn't stop myself' (2012: 93). Adams also draws on fight and military metaphors to describe the battle against his addiction: 'I was trying to run my life like a football match. I've lost today. Shit. Try to do better next time' (Adams, 1998: 17). Here, alcoholism is an illness to be fought, much as his opponents were, and 'winning' is being 'recovered'.

Returning to the notion of restitution, all four (auto)biographies draw on the fight metaphor to describe a comeback to their sport after periods in rehabilitation and treatments centres. Describing 30 days spent in the Betty Ford Centre, Daly writes that he 'came out of a Betty Ford a stronger human being ... My whole life right then was trying to get new sponsors and get back on the Tour' (2006: 100–102). Similarly, Kelly Smith describes a period spent at the Sporting Chance Clinic, a specialist rehabilitation centre set up by Tony Adams for sportsmen and women battling addictions: 'I had to recover before I could start thinking or dreaming about football again. I also had to get my spirit back so that I could start to want to do all those things again (2012: 103).

In other words, fight metaphors were closely connected to the desire to return to one's former life and sport. As Tony Adams writes: 'If I could bring myself to devote as much energy and enthusiasm to staying off the booze as I had to my football, then I had a chance. I had, after all, always been a winner in football' (1998: 22).

The journey

'Life is a journey'. This metaphor is readily overlaid on lives that have been fundamentally altered by illness or addiction. It is particularly applicable to alcoholism, where the experience of addiction may have been a part of an individual's life for many years, in some cases even decades. Metaphors of 'the journey' are evocative and convey the sense of a passage of time in which the journey continues through treatment and beyond. Smith, for example, describing her experiences in rehabilitation, writes that:

> it helps being helped by people who have been on a similar journey in their life. I would go so far as to say that I don't think I would have got the help I needed if those people hadn't been through what I had been through. This is an important part of it all. We could help each other out along the same path (2012: 104).

In the metaphor of the journey, the road or path may be bumpy and poorly sign-posted at times, and individuals may encounter crossroads or roadblocks along the way, but the language of 'moving on' or 'moving ahead' is consistent across the four (auto)biographies. Daly, for example, writes that 'I don't know what I'll do next, but I'll keep on keeping on. I don't like to live in the past, and I'm a little leery of predicting the future. I've done that too many times. By the time it finally gets here, and the future does turn into the present and bite me on the ass' (2006: 184). For each athlete addict, their 'journey' has a starting point or departure, with early life experiences featuring in the construction of the narrative of their book, with reaching the pinnacle of their sport being seen as the ultimate destination. The idea of a journey is also present in the language of recovery, where each of the (auto)biographies describes the process of rehabilitation as 'being on the road to recovery'.

Importantly, notions of place are an important theme in the journey. Each of the (auto)biographies describes starting out – 'growing up in Watford' (Smith, 2012: 1), or Essex (Adams, 1998), as a 'redneck kid in Arkansas' (Daly, 2008: 1) and as a 'Belfast man' (Higgins, 2000: 7) – and often in circumstances of social and material disadvantage. The narrative of the poor boy made good provided part of the backstory to the biography of Daly and Hurricane. Daly, for example, recalls that growing up in Arkansas that 'our family wasn't rich or anything' (2000: 18), while Higgins' account is littered with references to growing up around the Belfast shipyards. In both of these accounts in particular, their sporting prowess – as a golfer and snooker player respectively – provided a way out of the working class or the locational disadvantage of their childhoods.

While it is beyond the scope of this chapter, it is worth noting that these sporting (auto)biographies, in which determined drunkenness features heavily, point to a wider problem in the policy discourse on 'binge drinking'; namely the taken-for-granted assumptions that couple drinking to excess with young people in socio-economically deprived communities. While class relations, or more specifically, class differences are not easily unpacked (Winlow and Hall, 2006), 'six pints of lager or a bottle of champagne can produce a transgressive pharmacological and cultural nexus that is not class specific' (Hayward and Hobbs, 2007: 437). Nonetheless, such behaviour is portrayed by the media as almost the default setting for young people from particular class backgrounds.

The biographies, do however, raise the question of how to present the sporting achievements of John Daly or Alex Higgins (along with the likes of George Best and Paul Gasgoigne, among others) without valorising the drinking so central to their presentation of self to the communities still mired in the social disadvantage that these sportsmen managed to escape? While being handy with a football or a billiard cue has enabled young people to escape a particular kind of habitus, excessive drinking remains inextricably linked to both their old and new biographies. In other words, a more nuanced consideration of how drinking may play into aspirational sporting biographies needs to be included as part of rethinking drinking in sport.

Continuing the journey metaphor, for Adams and Smith in particular, their illness and subsequent treatment was seen as disrupting their sporting journey, throwing their lives into utter chaos. Adams, for example, recalls that 'when I had my football, I was all right, in control, focussed. In that state, I would look in the mirror and say to myself, "Right. Remember how you are now. Let's try and keep it". On other days, when I was drinking, I would look in the mirror and just wonder, "why can't you stop this now?"' (1998: 14). Similarly, Smith writes that counselling sessions in and after her time spent at the Sporting Chance clinic 'kept her grounded, focussed me on the job in hand, to get me through each week as well as help me set goals in terms of what I still wanted to achieve in my life' (2012: 105). Daly also recounts the chaotic nature of drinking, and its impact on his game:

> Basically, my golf in 1992 played second fiddle to making money and partying.
> Instead of partying I guess I ought to just say drinking, which is what it was. For
> the first time in my life, I let my golf game slide. That whole year, I don't, think
> I practiced more than two days in a row. And it showed (2006: 61).

In presenting the chaos of drinking, the (auto)biographies all capture the athlete's sense of a lost or fragmented identity during this time. Each of the biographies used language like 'falling apart emotionally' or 'struggling to keep myself together'. Describing an episode of self-harm, Smith, for example, recalls that 'it is not something I am proud of today. What more can I say? I was lost. I was scared. I didn't know who I was anymore' (2012: 102). Accordingly, emotions occupy a place of symbolic pre-eminence in the chaos narrative.

The return

Coming back once more to Frank's (1991) notion of the restitution narrative, the final stage is the return, where the owner of the story is no longer 'ill', but nonetheless remains marked by the illness. Smith writes that she 'managed to get off the drink, which was great. I was lucky. Today I can manage my drinking OK. I still drink sometimes, but in a controlled way. I still have to work on it though' (2012: 105). Similarly, Adams writes that:

> Today, I am not just Tony Adams the footballer, I am Tony Adams the human being. I do my best everyday on every walk of life and seek to treat myself and other people with respect. In that there is also victory. Winning on the field is sweet, of course, but in addition, as far as I'm concerned, with each day that I do not take a drink, I will always be a winner (1998: 258).

In his restitution narrative, Frank refers to the 'paradigmatic hero' who has 'travelled beyond, remains marked by illness and vows to return and share this with others' (1991: 84). Adams provides the example here. Following his own recovery, Adams established the Sporting Chance clinic, a specialist addiction and recovery facility for athletes that has subsequently treated athletes such as Kelly Smith.

A final aspect of the journey is convincing others that, through experience of illness and recovery from addiction, something has been gained; a new perspective on life, or an appreciation for what one has. Here, the illness of alcoholism is construed as offering 'life lessons'. Daly, for example, reflects that 'I just want Sherrie [wife] to understand that I'm doing what I'm doing for her and me and our kids' (2006: 190).

'Writing' Addiction through Cultural Scripts

Analytically then, the cultural scripts that are articulated in relation to the restitution narrative of an athlete's journey through and recovery from alcohol abuse also raises some important questions about the nature of addiction. If, as is widely accepted, alcoholism is a disease requiring a medical response, then what can be said about the agency and responsibility of the 'addict' in the context of elite sport? How can addicts make sense of this dimension of a multi-valenced life? Autobiographies, such as those presented here, I'd suggest, give voice and agency to the ways in which they author or 'script' their own stories of self. Smith, for example, recalls her experience in Alcoholics Anonymous where 'relating your problems to stories about other people's drinking and hearing how they coped and got through it was pretty powerful' (2012: 104). Such biographies, I'd argue, also challenge assumptions about the 'masculine, masterful, disciplined nature of elite sport', for all of the (auto)biographies described here also tell of an athlete who is 'physically compromised' (Sear and Fraser, 2010: 176) through their illness.

Notwithstanding the difficulties with attempting to define alcoholism described in Chapter 1, where its meaning is contested both within and between disciplines

(Poland and Graham, 2011), the cultural scripts presented here illustrate that addiction is neither a matter of an excessive 'liking' of drinking (Berridge and Robinson, 2011), nor is it simply a consequence of experimenting with addictive substances.[2] Indeed, alcoholics (and drug users) face a challenge of claiming and articulating a sense of self in the midst of a whole set of contradictory expectations about how they can, will and should perform these different selves against broader assumptions of what alcoholism is. Biographies and autobiographies, the evocative nature of metaphors and the cultural scripts that are written about the experience of addiction can provide important devices through which to narrate a story, a presentation and a performance of self. The stories of the addicts themselves, captured here in their biographies and autobiographies, suggests there is something powerful in being able to share one's story with an audience that as Adams put it 'may have suspected all along' (1996: 222).

Arguably, the ways in which athletes such as Kelly Smith or Tony Adams detail their experiences of recovery and rehabilitation as an 'athlete addict' emphasise the ways in which telling one's story can act as a therapeutic tool. Drawing on the ideas of cultural scripts and media framings, it is possible, once the story of addiction and recovery has been told, to then examine the form of the story (its structure or its plot) and its content (what happened) in order to provide lessons and strategies for the recovery of others.

Stories of Place

As I outlined at the start of the chapter, a key dimension in biographies of drinking is the notion of 'place', and the stories that accompany drinking environments; that is, where people drink, where they grew up and, in some cases, where they learned to drink. Equally, the affective dimensions of place; that is, of 'being in a bad place' when or because of drinking were part of the cultural scripts described in this chapter. I will tease out some of the cultural scripts through which these stories of place are narrated shortly, but it is necessary to locate them within a consideration of the geographies of drinking more broadly that, conceptually, underpins this section.

Geographies of Drinking

Geographers such as Mark Jayne and Gil Valentine have noted that the relationships between the people, practices and processes of drinking and drunkenness and the places where people are drinking and getting drunk are becoming increasingly important topics of inquiry (Jayne, et al., 2008a; 2008b). Similarly, Measham argues that 'research on drugs, leisure and spatiality intersects with some of the

---

2 Most people who use "potentially addicting substances do not become addicts, but between 15% and 17% do" (Morse, 2011:176).

most interesting recent debate in cultural criminology, cultural geography and cultural studies' (2004b: 337). Most of the research on drugs, leisure and spatiality however, has been done in terms of fun and hedonism, rather than the spatial relations to alcoholism that I will discuss shortly.

As described in Chapter 2, drinking and drunkenness are key components of backpacking holidays, shaping the rhythm of travel through the spatial and temporal imperatives of 'passing the time' and 'being able to do nothing', as well as heightening a sense of belonging with both fellow travellers and the 'locals' they encounter in bars, pubs, clubs and the like (Jayne, et al., 2012: 211), and softening a number of (un)comfortable embodied and emotional materialities associated with budget travel (i.e. lumpy dormitory beds), all of which become 'stories to tell'. In their analysis of drinking stories amongst Danish youth in the Bulgarian resort of Sunny Beach, Tutenges and Sandberg (2013) similarly argue that the stories young people recount of drinking and partying are part of their stock of future storytelling capital. Tutenges and Sandberg (2013) suggest that there may be a constitutive relationship between storytelling and social action so that the stories they tell of drunken transgressions are a key part of the holiday experience and the representation by these young people of having fun and being young. Similarly, in her discussion of the après-ski culture of snowboarding, Thorpe notes that 'the hedonistic behaviours of participants in bars, nightclubs and other cultural spaces have gone largely ignored' (2012: 34). As Jayne, et al., (2012), Tutenges and Sandberg (2013) and Thorpe (2012) all recognise, the extent (and limits) of pleasure, in *spatial* terms, as well as in social terms, discussed earlier in the book, is key to understanding the cultural drivers which underpin drinking practices.

Certainly, much of the material presented in the book so far engages, although not directly, with the spatial dimensions of alcohol consumption. Jayne, et al., provide a useful summary that reflects the broad interests of the book so far:

> Research has addressed a large number of diverse topics relating to legislation, policy and policing, production, marketing and retail, consumption, identity, lifestyle and forms of sociability (and so on) at transnational, national, regional and local spatial scales. Indeed, a key feature of these studies has been a concern with "geographical" issues such as spatial scale, boundaries and transgressions; distinctions between public and private, visibility and invisibility, centrality and marginality, urbanity and rurality, and so on (2008a: 249).

While a large body of research has attempted to identify the ways in which issues related to alcohol, drinking and drunkenness unfold in specific spaces and places – research into the night time economy, for example, including; the numbers, density and types of outlets; the design and layout of venues; server intervention (relating to age and levels of intoxication), and the impacts of levels and types of law enforcement (see Plant, et al., 2001) – far less attention has been paid to the role of 'place' in constructing the biographies of *drinkers* that I am interested in here. As I discuss in the following section, space and place are not 'passive backdrops' to drinking but are active constituents in the practices and experiences bound up with alcohol consumption.

To more explicitly interrogate the spatial dimensions of sport-based drinking, the chapter returns to the (auto)biographies of drinking and the stories of place that frame much of the cultural scripts that orient the texts. The 'place' of drinking (and drunkenness) is discussed in relation to two key sites of drinking – the pub/ nightclub and the home. The emotional aspects of drinking – of 'being in a bad place' when or because of drinking – are also discussed.

Places of Drinking: Public Drinking

As has been well documented in the literature, pubs and nightclubs have been key social spaces in the leisure pursuits of young adults in countries such as Australia, New Zealand or the United Kingdom. While the sociality of drinking has been addressed elsewhere in the book, it is the spatiality of drinking that this chapter is more principally concerned with. In the pub and club, there is a clear relationship between spatiality, consumption and commercial imperatives. In most urban areas, vertical, large-capacity establishments used mostly for the sale and consumption of alcohol (and also illicit drug-taking), which offer little or no seating for their patrons are among the more prominent spatial features of the night-time economy. Along with pubs, including sports bars and theme pubs (e.g. Australiana pubs such as the 'Walkabout' chain or traditional British pubs transplanted into the south of Spain), these nightclubs have long served as environments in which calculated hedonism and determined drunkenness can be enacted and embodied. As I address later in the chapter, the public nature of drinking in these establishments can also make maximally visible a person's problematic relationships to alcohol. Indeed, it is frequently during a night of intoxication at a pub or club where images and narratives of a drunken athlete as a 'fool or a villain' emerge (Lines, 2001).

In terms of sport-related drinking, the pub (public house) has long served as an important socio-spatial site. In other writings relating to the history of sport in Britain, scholars Richard Holt (1990) and Wray Vamplew (1988) refer to a timeless and yet fluid bond that is shared between the pub and sport. More recently Kraszewski (2008) and Dixon (2011) indicate that going to the pub (including sports bars and theme pubs) has become part of routine practice for millions of fans worldwide. Weed (2006) has similarly shown that even when pubs (in the United Kingdom) showing major football matches are not serving alcohol (such as outside normal licensing hours), supporters can still turn the watching of the match into a significant social event through singing and chanting and other forms of social performing. Following on from this, Dixon (2014) examines the relationships that fans of English football have with the pub or what he terms 'an enduring site for fandom practice' (2014; 382). His findings suggest that fans have an important, emotive connection to the pub as a 'football space, one that is associated sociability and the perception of cultural stability' (Dixon, 2014: 382).

To return to the biographies of drinking, pubs and nightclubs featured heavily in the cultural scripts that the athletes presented. Unlike the construction of the sport-pub nexus as one of camaraderie and bonding between fans, in the accounts of Tony Adams and Kelly Smith in particular, the pub is a highly contradictory drinking environment; that is, a space of social interaction and solitary drinking. As Adams recounts: 'I was always assured of sympathy and company at my local … ' (1998: 210). Continuing this notion of the pub or club as a site and source of social interaction, Adams recalls:

> When live Sunday football was introduced, it gave me an excuse to stay down the pub all day. On Sundays I would either move on from my starting point of The Chequers or I would find other little pubs and clubs … We would do a few social or Irish clubs … then I discovered Ra Ra's, the nightclub in Islington where I met Jane [Adams' former wife], and I had somewhere cheerful to go on those gloomy Sunday nights. This is rocking, this'll do for me, I remember thinking (1998: 203).

Alongside such accounts of sociality, both Adams and Smith remember the pub as a place without interaction, where they could 'just be left alone to drink' (Smith, 2012: 45). Adams describes an early morning visit to a pub on his way to a training session: 'I only had two pints in The Chequers, just to take the edge off, to settle my stomach. Nobody said anything to me. Typical alcoholic that, I have come to realise' (1998: 211). Smith, similarly, describes an aborted return to training camp following a period of injury: 'I see a sign for a Harvester pub and I don't think about what to do next. I park the car, walk into the bar and order myself a couple of vodkas, then a couple more. I set about drinking myself into oblivion. I'm alone' (2012: 8).

Yet, even if drinking alone, the inherently public dimensions of a pub or club means that the solitary drinking, the altercations, the scrapes with the bouncers and the refusals of service that pepper both Adams and Smith's autobiographies are played out publicly. As noted earlier, it is frequently during a night of intoxication at a pub or club where images and narratives of a drunken athlete as a 'fool or a villain' (Lines, 2001) emerge, a theme echoed by Adams, in particular: 'there have been the public episodes, like falling down nightclub steps and having 20 stitches inserted in my head' (1998: 19).

Places of Drinking: Domestic Drinking

Alongside the pub, the home featured in the accounts of Adams' and Smiths' accounts of drinking. The domestic home, the marital home, homes away from home, such as training camps, dormitories and shared college rooms, were among the drinking places acknowledged in their (auto)biographies. That the home (and related domestic spaces) feature in accounts of drinking recognises a broader shift in drinking patterns that is being acknowledged in the literature more broadly. As I return to in Chapter 8, the increasing availability of relatively cheap alcohol through supermarkets, along with bottle shops with extended opening hours have changed the drinking landscape and, as I discuss in this section, these have been important in facilitating home drinking, particularly practices such as 'pre-loading' (i.e. getting drunk before leaving home for a night out) or simply 'loading' at home, as Smith's and Adams' accounts both attest to.

Despite 'domestic drinking' or home drinking becoming increasingly common practice, and in many cases socially sanctioned and normalised (Holloway, Jayne and Valentine, 2008), its socially accepted and acceptable status means that it has hovered on the margins of academic and policy interest. Concerns with public safety, violence, fatalities and injuries that are often part of the discourse around pubs, clubs and the night-time economy has meant that the 'problem' of drinking has been focused on the city centre. Following Holloway, Jayne and Valentine, I contend that:

> Contemporary public and policy debate about alcohol, which centres on these questions of regeneration and fears of drunken disorder, is overly biased towards particular conceptions of problem drinking in public space, and that there is an urgent need to consider the nature and importance of drinking in the domestic sphere (2008: 532).

Indeed, it is interesting to note that while most political and media attention has focused on the city centre, drinking at home is a relatively neglected but significant part of the market. Holloway, Jayne and Valentine (2008: 534) note that in Britain alone, 54 per cent of British adults in 2011 had a drink at home at least once a week, compared with only 28 per cent who did so outside the home (Mintel 2004), while the off-licence trade in Britain accounts for 49 per cent of drink sold in terms of volume (Mintel 2005). In other words, despite the increasing popularity of it as a social practice, the 'relative silence about home drinking in public debate is reproduced in academia where comparatively little has been written about it within the geographical and wider social science literature' (Holloway, Jayne and Valentine, 2008: 534).

However, as both Adams' and Smith's (auto)biographies make clear, domestic drinking provides a space where alcohol intake can exceed government guidelines without the scrutiny of the public gaze. Similarly, Daly recalls his family garage as being a place 'where Dad liked to go to drink' (2000: 29). For both Smith and Adams, the home (or living spaces such as college dormitories or hotel bedrooms) was where drinking started and continued, and where acts of regret and remorse were committed. Adams, for example, recalls the shame of home drinking: 'then there was the stuff I managed to keep private; frequently wetting the bed' (1998: 19), while Smith describes 'while sitting at home in my apartment alone, drinking by myself, those thoughts in my head got worse and worse' (2012: 94).

The solitary and hidden nature of domestic drinking, described, here, unlike widespread, socially sanctioned practices such as wine with dinner, means that harmful domestic 'binge' drinking, unlike public binge drinking can escape public scrutiny, masking the extent of the kinds of problematic relationships to alcohol described in this chapter.

Finally, along with the physical locations of the pub or the home as drinking spaces, affective references were made to drinking, space and place where 'place' became an emotive site. Geographical references such as being 'in a bad place' when drinking, being at 'rock bottom' and being 'in a fog' when drinking were common in the (auto)biographies of Smith and Adams in particular. Unlike the pleasure of drinking, which casts the interplay between emotions, space, place, drinking and drunkenness in particular ways, the intersection of emotion, alcohol and addiction presents a very different 'interpretive framing' (Silverman, 2013) of the narrative of drinking and drunkenness. Here, emotions are 'embodied and mindful phenomena that partially shape, and are shaped by our interaction with people, places and politics that make up our unique, personal geographies' (Davidson and Bondi, 2004: 373).

Conclusion

This chapter has been concerned with some of the narratives of alcohol 'addiction' among professional and elite level athletes, particularly their 'fall from grace', their decline, recovery and, in some cases, their death. Drawing on four key (auto)biographies that tell the story of an athlete's struggle with addiction, the chapter has examined some of the contradictory themes or fault lines that run through the particular construction and presentation of narratives of addiction in professional sport. Drawing on Frank's (1991) notion of the restitution narrative, the (auto)biographies point to C. Wright Mills' reminder that biography and history intersect, and that neither 'the life of the individual nor the history of a society could be understood without understanding both' (1959: 3). Analytically then, the interest of this chapter was with a life history of drinking; of how alcohol is written into (and out of) the lives of sportsmen and women. As I have described here, biographies and autobiographies, the evocative nature of metaphors, and the cultural scripts that are written about the experience of addiction also provide important devices through which to narrate a presentation of self. The stories of the addicts themselves, captured in their biographies and autobiographies, suggest there is something powerful in being able to share one's 'restitution narrative' with an audience.

The chapter was also interested in the role and importance of 'place' in the construction and articulation of these biographies of drinking in sport. As Jayne, et al. note 'drinking and drunkenness can be understood as patterns of activities that take on different meanings within a constellation of interlocking practices performed by people who simultaneously shape places and are shaped by places' (2008b: 214).

The chapter also provides the segue to the second half of the book– *Tackling the Problem* – which focuses on the implications of the kinds of behaviours and practices discussed in this first half for policy and practice. The chapters in this second section deal primarily with the relationships between sport, alcohol, prevention and rehabilitation, where sport provides a setting for a number of programmes aimed at the prevention of, or recovery from, alcohol-related abuses. As I discuss in the following chapter, there are a range of strategies and initiatives that sporting clubs and communities have put in place to address, recognise, challenge and change the 'culture of drinking' in sport.

PART II
Tackling the Problem

Chapter 6
Changing the Culture

This chapter:
- examines some of the initiatives and interventions by sporting clubs and communities to address the 'culture of drinking' in sport;
- reviews the relative success and limitations of various initiatives intended to reduce or mitigate some of the social and health harms of sport-related drinking;
- explores the role of lay knowledge and lay strategies in keeping drinkers safe.

Introduction

This first chapter in this second section moves away from questions of identity, drinking cultures and communities, and the relationships that sportsmen and women have to alcohol that were discussed in previous chapters, and begins to look at some of the strategies, initiatives and interventions that sporting clubs and the communities in which they are located have put in place to address, recognise, change and challenge the 'culture of drinking' in sport. As I elaborate in this chapter, community-based sporting clubs are often sites of unregulated problematic and unsafe drinking, yet at the same time many clubs have attempted, with various degrees of success, to address the costs and consequences of this. In light of the material presented earlier in the book, arguments for culture change raise several key issues and questions for sociological studies of sport, in particular, how do we reconcile the tensions between the pleasure of calculated hedonism or determined drunkenness and the criminal or illegal behaviour that many culture change initiatives have been developed to respond to?

Building on the material introduced in previous chapters, this chapter reviews and critiques the relative success and limitations of various initiatives intended to reduce or mitigate some of the social and health harms of sport-related drinking. Formal interventions such as the Good Sports programme or the Play Hard, Drink Safe programme, both from Australia, or the introduction of family friendly areas that are differentiated from designated drinking areas at sporting grounds and venues, through to more informal initiatives adopted and implemented by drinkers and patrons themselves will be reviewed. In other words, the concern of this chapter is to draw together the preceding empirical research to argue for an approach to sport-related drinking that can promote responsibility and sociality at one and the same time. As I argue in what follows, there is some evidence that the *formal* interventions implemented by clubs have proven to be quite ineffectual in encouraging responsible alcohol consumption, with some of the more effective strategies often being operationalised at an *informal* level by drinkers and patrons themselves. As I suggest in the following pages, drinkers are actively engaged in a range of creative, 'lay' strategies that seek to minimise the harmful consequences of their own – and others' – drinking. While the focus of the chapter is on sport, the key arguments developed are of relevance to those engaged in health promotion and behaviour change research and education more broadly.

In terms of how the chapter unfolds, three key initiatives adopted by sporting clubs are discussed, followed by a consideration of the effectiveness of their safe alcohol policies and other in-club strategies to reduce the sale and consumption of alcohol. While the focus is on football (Australian Rules and rugby league) this is not to suggest that it is only football where a culture of intoxication prevails and where culture change initiatives have been implemented. The 'Know When to Declare' campaign launched in 2009 by Cricket Australia suggests anecdotal cause for concern within that sport. To date however, there is not an established evidential base as evidence of its uptake by cricket spectators. Thus research on football, and from Australia, provides the focus for this chapter.

The Context

In Australia alone approximately 4.5 million Australians are involved in community sports clubs, and a high level of alcohol consumption tends to be commonplace in this setting. Despite many commendable policy initiatives that seek to regulate and moderate the sale, purchase and consumption of alcohol at sporting clubs and venues, some of which are discussed shortly, sports-associated drinking remains a persistent problem. As Duff and Munro note 'this culture is manifested in ritual binge drinking, the use of alcohol as rewards for sporting performances, and end-of-season trips that resemble a drinking safari. Offensive behaviour, physical and relational violence, assaults and drunk driving have been accepted as collateral damage' (2007: 1992). Geoff Munro, the national policy manager for the Australian Drug Foundation (cited in Kelly, Hickey, et al.) claims that 'sports/clubs have known of player "drinking incidents" (whatever they may be) for many years, but have turned a blind eye … They can no longer do so. I think the public is demanding a higher standard of behaviour, and sports are only going to miss out if administrators don't take action' (2011: 467).

Certainly, there is a tendency to imagine sports clubs as spaces in which alcohol plays a significant and unequivocally problematic role, and research suggests there is strong community support to break the (community) sport-alcohol nexus. In their survey of community attitudes in Victoria, Tobin, Fitzgerald, et al. (2012), found that there was widespread support for structural alterations to the drinking context, such as removing alcohol sponsorship of community sport and imposing a levy on alcohol advertising. This was particularly the case among women, older-aged and non-English-speaking citizens and those not involved in sport clubs.

Organisational difficulties, however, compound the problem of harmful levels of alcohol consumption within sporting clubs. Many clubs depend on volunteer staff who typically lack training in the responsible service of alcohol and many clubs rely on the sale of alcohol as a reliable source of revenue. Many clubs hold a restricted or limited liquor license that allows them to serve alcohol during designated hours on designated days: usually they are restricted to match days, during and after training, and at special functions. However, as Duff and Munro note 'clubs have a financial incentive to maximize the amount of alcohol they sell and it is common for officials to ignore licensing regulations in the interest of generating funds and providing a "sociable" atmosphere' (2007: 1992). Following on from this, Kingsland, Wolfenden, et al. (2013) argue that risky consumption is more likely to occur in small clubs and where alcohol is served to intoxicated people, during happy hour promotions (i.e. where alcohol is provided at a discounted rate for a defined period of time) and where alcohol-only awards or prizes are given out, finding that members of clubs where these practices take place are more than twice as likely to consume alcohol to excess.

Emerging as a significant social problem that implicates drink driving, sexual assault, violence, malicious damage, relationship difficulties, unsafe sex, financial issues and absenteeism (AIHW, 2011), a number of interventions have been developed within and for sporting clubs that are aimed, primarily, at reducing the health and social impacts of intoxication. Ranging from large-scale government policy initiatives such as the Good Sports programme in Australia, which seeks systematic behaviour change in sporting clubs; to the Alcohol Management Operation in New Zealand, which adopts a harm minimisation approach; or the Choose Life Choose Sports programme operating in Macedonia, which advocates the use of safe drinking champions to promote responsible drinking among young sportsmen and women; through to more targeted legislation to regulate or ban the advertising or purchase of alcohol at sporting venues (particularly where children and young people are present), such initiatives weave together a range of health and social policy concerns that are explored in the following pages.

The Good Sports Programme

In Australia, the most comprehensive policy initiative is the Good Sports programme. Funded by the federal government through the Australian Drug Foundation, the Good Sports programme – believed to be only programme of its type in the world – was developed in 2001 in response to a perceived escalation in the costs and consequences of harmful drinking within sporting clubs (ADF, 2002; Munro, 2000; 2007). Triggered by the death of a young Australian Rules footballer in regional Victoria following an extended post-match drinking session with his teammates, the Good Sports programme encourages sporting clubs (including cricket, netball and surf lifesaving as well as Australian Rules, soccer and rugby) to monitor and manage the sale and consumption of alcohol on their premises, particularly with regard to underage and 'binge' drinking.

The broad intentions of the Good Sports programme are for clubs to gain accreditation in the responsible service of alcohol and to minimise their dependency on alcohol sales to finance club activities. As I'll return to however, despite clubs imagining and implementing an impressive range of strategies designed to manage alcohol consumption, many of the cultural practices associated with 'binge' or heavy episodic drinking are ones that some club members gain pleasure from as 'calculated hedonists' (see Chapter 2) and this presents a considerable challenge to club policies that seek to unilaterally discourage intoxication within the club.

Supported by an above and below the line media campaign including television and radio advertisements, in-venue posters and drinks coasters, the fundamental tenet of the Good Sports programme is one of culture change, in which the behaviours and practices of sporting clubs – and their patrons – are subject to a certain degree of surveillance and normative peer pressure. Reducing the incidence or frequency of sport-related drinking by discouraging it as a *club* activity, rather than minimising the harms attached to drinking by individuals underpins the strategic policy focus of the Good Sports programme.

Play Hard, Drink Safe

Using the basic premises of the Good Sports programme as a starting point, several states and territories in Australia and elsewhere have adopted similar, scaled down versions of the programme to encourage safer levels of drinking as the cultural norm within their sporting clubs and communities. In Western Australia, for example, the Western Australian Health Promotion Foundation (Healthway) has initiated a pilot sponsorship project in five sporting clubs aimed at promoting responsible alcohol consumption. For a large state – encompassing 2,529,875 kilometres; the entire western third of Australia – much of Western Australia's population live in regional and remote communities where problematic drinking remains a pernicious social problem more broadly. In particular, drink driving is a key issue, with taxis and police drug and alcohol testing units scarce so drinkers are more likely to 'chance their arm' on getting home without getting caught. At the same time, sporting clubs in rural and regional towns operate as 'communities of interest' (Winter, 2000) that provide and develop social connections and civic participation in ways that contribute to the emotional, social and mental health of many remote and rural settings (Tonts, 2005). Indeed, at a community level, 'sporting clubs do much more than simply promote physical activity and participation in sport. They also serve as social meeting places in which individuals develop a sense of shared values and beliefs' (Kelly, Hickey et al., 2011: 4689). Schemes such as Play Hard, Drink Safe attempt to chart the middle waters between responsibility and sociality.

The Play Hard, Drink Safe programme was one of several transactional schemes introduced by Healthway. Established in 1991 under tobacco control legislation that banned tobacco sponsorship, Healthway offers sponsorship to 'arts, sports and racing organisations in exchange for the promotion of health messages at sponsored events and the implementation of healthy environment policies in sponsored venues, notably smoke-free policies' (Clarkson, Giles-Corti, et al., 2002: 227).

Five sporting clubs in Western Australia (bowling, rugby, tennis and two general sport and recreation clubs) received Healthway sponsorship of between AUD$3,000 and AUD$5,000 to promote the message: 'Play Hard, Drink Safe (PHDS)'. Clubs were required to:

- promote low and mid-strength tap beers, and provide a price incentive on lower-strength beers;
- implement server training in responsible alcohol service;
- display an 'Accord' carrying the PHDS message in the bar area (informing members that the bar staff had been trained in responsible alcohol service and that the club policy was to refuse to serve alcohol to intoxicated patrons);
- display a range of promotional materials carrying the PHDS sponsorship message, such as beer mats, table signs, posters and promotional clothing for bar staff;
- run special PHDS promotional evenings at intervals during the sponsorship period, such as competitions and low alcohol beer tastings; and implement smoke-free policies in indoor club rooms (a standard requirement in all Healthway sponsorships (Clarkson, Giles-Corti, et al., 2002: 227).

Post-intervention interviews were conducted with bar managers to assess the implementation of responsible serving practices, the perceived impact of the sponsorship on sales of alcoholic and non-alcoholic drinks and patron attitudes to responsible alcohol consumption in the clubs.

While there were reasonable levels of recall of the Play Hard, Drink Safe message, the scheme, perhaps surprisingly, appeared to have little impact on alcohol consumption in the clubs. Both the pre- and post-intervention measures similarly reported that more than 50 per cent of respondents recounted consuming more than the recommended safe alcohol limits in their club. Sales of reduced strength beers did not increase and price incentives did not have any impact on beer sales (Clarkson, Giles-Corti, et al., 2002: 227). While it is not my intention here to answer it, the perceived limitations of this scheme to reduce harmful levels of alcohol consumption within the pilot clubs raises the question of context, and the broader setting within which the drinking occurs which makes determined drunkenness both enjoyable and expected, and makes it difficult for such initiatives to find traction.

While the Good Sports and the Play Hard, Drink Safe programmes operated within a framework of social marketing, broad culture change and awareness raising, other schemes operate from the perspective of harm minimisation or of 'doing things a little less dangerously'. The Alcohol Management Operation is a case in point.

Alcohol Management Operation

The Alcohol Management Operation [AMO] was developed in New Zealand and it adopts a harm minimisation approach to sport-related drinking. Instigated by 'street level bureaucrats' (Lipsky, 1980) such as emergency rescue teams exasperated at being called out to deal with patrons who had been killed or injured in motor vehicle accidents following drinking sessions at their sports club, the AMO explicitly acknowledges the potentially health damaging behaviours of sport-related drinking, and the sheer inevitability with which they will occur. With its strapline of 'Plan for Getting Plastered', the AMO seeks not so much to challenge in-club drinking practices but to 'do them a little less dangerously'. The AMO recognises that drinking to the point of intoxication cannot, in and of itself, be discouraged. What *can* be moderated however, are its consequences, through 'plans for getting plastered' such as nominating the designated driver or agreeing the time to depart a venue *before* settling in for a session at the club.

Anecdotal evidence also attests to a number of more informal initiatives being instigated by clubs and coaches (in both Australia and New Zealand), such as restricting post-match drinking to non-alcoholic beverages until after a player has urinated, encouraging the purchase of food alongside alcohol when buying drinks, distancing the service of alcohol from junior time slots and social activities, and discouraging 'all you can drink' entry tickets to club social functions.

While targeted schemes that deal directly with the use of sport to deter young people from poor life choices (such as crime or alcohol misuse) are discussed in the following chapter, the examples of the Good Sports programme, the Drink Hard, Play Safe pilot programme and the Alcohol Management Operation provide useful case studies from which to begin to interrogate questions of evidence and effectiveness with this and similar culture change programmes.

Assessment of the Solution and Strategies

Despite these and other initiatives that seek to regulate and moderate the sale, purchase and consumption of alcohol at sporting clubs and venues, sports-associated drinking remains a persistent problem, which suggests not only a need to question the effectiveness of such initiatives, but also to question the assumptions on and the tools through which measures of effectiveness are determined. In the context of increasing spending cuts, a global economic downturn, and public scrutiny and accountability for the deliverables of sports policy, the issues for evidence-based and evidence-informed policy-making are particularly important.

While there appears to be no evaluation of the Alcohol Management Operation and, as indicated earlier, the evaluation of the Drink Hard, Play Safe pilot suggested limited success in terms of behaviour change around safe alcohol consumption, evaluations of the Good Sports programme consistently conclude that it has been effective in bringing about incremental rather than wholesale culture change within community-based sporting clubs. Rowland, Allen and Toumbourou (2012a; 2012b), for example, sought to examine the association of risky alcohol consumption with the level of accreditation of a club in the Good Sports programme. Drawing on a cross section of football and cricket clubs, multilevel modelling indicated that higher accreditation in the Good Sports programme by a club is associated with reduced rates of risky alcohol use at a population level.

Similarly, Crundall (2012) examined the extent to which improved alcohol management in clubs where the Good Sports programme was in place delivered any additional benefits to clubs, such as financial viability through revenue sources other than alcohol sales or an expanded membership base. Crundall's research, based on survey information collected prior to clubs receiving Level 1 accreditation and at their third and final level of club accreditation, found that income increased and a reliance on alcohol as a funding source diminished over time.[1] Membership increased, particularly among women, young people and non-players. No changes in the number of junior and senior teams or players were found. In other words, in this case, improved alcohol management seemed to produce a range of benefits beyond responsible drinking behaviours that added to club sustainability (Crundall, 2012).

Both of these evaluations suggest that the Good Sports programme is a model of modest incremental change employed by community sporting clubs in the interest of eliminating harmful drinking practices and establishing safer norms of use *over time*. Issues of time and scale however, suggest caution for isolating the Good Sports programme as an effective behaviour change scheme from other factors that are indirectly or not at all related to the incremental intervention. Leaver-Dunn, Turner and Newman (2007), for example, assessed the ways in which recreational activities in the United States that were undertaken by young men could positively influence young men's use of alcohol and their intentions to consume alcohol. They found that there were protective effects of involvement in recreational activities on alcohol abuse and intentions but no effect on engagement

---

1 The Good Sports Accreditation Levels can be summarised as follows: **Level 1:** Liquor license; Bar management strategies; Responsible Service of Alcohol (RSA) training; Smoke-free environment. **Level 2:** Maintain Level 1 standards; Enhanced bar management (RSA training, etc.); Food and drink options (low and non-alcoholic); Safe transport policy; Diverse revenue generation. **Level 3:** Maintain Level 1 and 2 standards. Alcohol management policy. Sporting clubs that do not serve or consume alcohol may still participate in Good Sports by registering in an alternative Level 0 program. **Level 0 Focus Areas:** Alcohol-free facilities; Smoke-free environment; Promotion of Good Sports; Safe transport policy (from http://goodsports.com.au/about/the-program/#sthash.QqPQBUwM.dpuf).

in sports activities, identifying that law enforcement and road safety initiatives had also been implemented in the United States at the time their research was undertaken. Accordingly, they recommended that studies that can successfully address these relationships may enhance the development of multi-dimensional interventions for reducing and preventing risk behaviours among young people (Leaver-Dunn, Turner and Newman, 2007).

Intervention Chains and Frameworks for Analysis

On the importance of multi-dimensional interventions, the work of the UK policy methodologist, Ray Pawson (2006) is instructive. Pawson and Tilley contend that 'intervention chains are long and thickly populated. Interventions carry not one, but several mechanisms of action' (2004: 5). In other words, when evaluating the effectiveness of particular interventions, it is often difficult to separate out which aspects of the intervention contribute to its effectiveness. Indeed, as Rowland, Allen and Toumbourou (2012a) acknowledge in relation to their evaluation of the Good Sports programme, developing prevention-focused interventions in these settings can be complex (Rowland, Allen and Toumbourou, 2012b) and there is a need to consider programmes in their broadest social context. As Pawson, et al. (2004: 7) contend,

> It is through the workings of entire systems of social relationships that any changes in behaviours, events and social conditions are effected. ... Rarely if ever is the 'same' programme equally effective in all circumstances because of the influence of contextual factors (2004: 7).

In the case of the Good Sports programme and the AMO, sport-related drinking does not always occur in the sporting clubs within which initiatives like Good Sports operate. Sport-related drinking takes place at sports grounds, in private homes, in nightclubs, and in other public spaces, where the consumption of alcohol falls beyond the governing gaze of a sporting club. That is, sport-related drinking occurs in people's homes, in pubs and hotels, and in other locations outside of the governing gaze of the 'charismatic cops, patriarchs and a few good women' that Kelly, et al. (2011) identify as being crucial figures in managing alcohol within sporting clubs.

Considering the broader cultural and spatial contexts within which sport-related drinking occurs is important, for not every sporting (football or otherwise) club has signed up to the Good Sports programme. Many sporting clubs are not signatories to the Good Sports programme; and, equally, among clubs that have signed up to the code of conduct around responsible alcohol management, determined drunkenness persists. Here, I'd suggest that the fun, enjoyment and pleasure gained from participating in drinking practices of the kind described in Chapter 2, and the normative pressure that keeps such traditions alive through the endless cycle of gearing up for, participating in, winding down from, then preparing again for the next drinking session, may outweigh any desire of the club to engage with the broader culture change agenda of initiatives like the Good Sports programme. Here the pleasure of drinking as a cultural practice obscures policy intent. As Harrison, et al. note, 'pleasure is silenced and or deployed strategically in neo-liberal governance discourses about drugs and alcohol … which raises questions about the limits of such discourses to affect changes in drinking patterns' (2011: 469).

Considering context and the long and thickly populated intervention chains highlights the need for evaluations and determinations of programme effectiveness to move beyond the 'black box' (Scriven, 1994) view much loved by policy makers, namely that traditional short-term sports programmes can effectively change a range of values, attitudes and behaviours, with little understanding of the processes through which this may or may not be achieved. Here, the realist evaluation approach of Pawson and Tilley (2004) can help penetrate the complexities of the intervention chains that run through programmes like Good Sports or the AMO.

In essence, realist evaluations, drawn from Critical Realism theory, argue for a need to evaluate programmes and policies in terms of their social and political context as well as the nuts and bolts of the programme itself. In other words, realist evaluation techniques recognise that there are many interwoven variables operating at different levels in society, that interventions can be complex, and very rarely is the 'traditional cause-effect, non-contextual evaluation of outcomes a particularly robust mechanism through which to make determinations about the effectiveness of a program' (Pawson and Tilley, 2004: 2). Looking to context as well as mechanistic considerations of what a programme is or does demands a reframing of the starting point for evaluations of these or similar programmes. As Pawson and Tilley note, we need to ask not 'what works' or 'does the program work', but ask instead 'what works, for whom in what respects and how' (2004: 2).

In asking questions about what works, in what ways and in what contexts, we return to questions of agency, and the relationships that are operationalised by drinkers themselves when making determinations on the outcomes of determined drunkenness. As I discuss below, drinkers are enormously adept at drawing on their own 'lay knowledge' to actively engage in a range of simple, 'mundane' strategies that seek to minimise the harmful consequences of their own – and others' – drinking. While it has been my intention to problematise, rather than answer questions of evidence and effectiveness in relation to formal programmes like the AMO or the Good Sports programme, empirical research suggests that informal strategies that draw on 'lay' knowledge that are adopted and implemented by drinkers and patrons themselves have a degree of direct effectiveness in ways that the intervention chain of a formal programme makes difficult to capture.

'Lay' Knowledge and Informal Strategies

Since the early part of this century there has been a growing interest in 'lay' knowledge in making choices about health damaging and health promoting behaviours. As Lupton argues 'lay' risk assessments and risk behaviours are often appropriate in the context of a person's life (1999). This valuing of lay knowledge recognises that the life experiences of 'ordinary' people provides them with a stock of knowledge through which to make decisions, and this often sits in opposition to expert, 'scientific' discourses on health behaviours, in this case, decisions around when, what, how and how much to drink.

This notion of lay knowledge has been discussed by Popay, et al. (2003), who uses it to describe the meanings given to, among other things, health and illness, that are influenced by the social circumstances in which people live. Here, lay knowledge and lay theories (sometimes known as 'lay epidemiology') (Davidson, et al., 1996) have been particularly illuminating in terms of better understanding people's views on health inequalities and health outcomes (Popay, et al., 2003). Elsewhere, Coveney, in his study of socio-economic differences in parental knowledge of food and nutrition, notes that 'lay knowledge is now regarded as significant in its own right and not merely a set of "quaint" beliefs subordinate to expertise or "scientific" knowledge' (2004: 294). For both Popay, et al. (2003) and Coveney (2004), lay knowledge is used to highlight the importance of one's own experiences in countering official or 'top down' messages around health promoting and health damaging behaviours.

In the same way, drinkers draw on their lay knowledge about drinking responsibly and irresponsibly to better understand the social context in which the meanings they attach to alcohol consumption and health promotion are constructed. In doing so, they operationalise key strategies that correspond to the broad analytical categories of 'keeping safe', 'minimising damage' and 'taking charge'. To illustrate this argument empirically, I return to the case study of Australian Rules football that I have referred to elsewhere in the book.

Informal Strategies

The methodological context has been described earlier in the book. In terms of lay knowledge and informal strategies, analysis of the interview data suggests that these strategies corresponded to three broad analytical themes: 'keeping safe'; 'minimising damage'; and 'taking charge', a similar pattern of analysis to that developed by Renker (2003) in relation to her work on adolescents keeping themselves safe from perinatal violence.

Keeping safe
The first theme, 'keeping safe', included narratives of mateship, rules on personal alcohol consumption and restrictions on drinking and driving. Mateship, in particular, featured heavily in respondents' accounts of their strategies for keeping safe:

> If I've seen people that are intoxicated and have a car I've found alternate transport for them or I've said "hey mate you're not driving home tonight, leave

your car here, put your keys in behind the bar, come and collect it tomorrow".
You look out for one another, you look after your mates (22-year-old male fan
of the southern suburbs club).

Elsewhere, fans alluded to the importance of mates overriding the decisions and
actions of an intoxicated other, as Bill, a fan of the western suburbs club describes:
'what's wrong with the old fashioned idea of looking after your mates? Like when
you see your mate's had one too many, I'll say, "mate, pull your head in, you've
had enough"'. In a related vein, respondents spoke of the dynamics of SANFL
themselves as contributing to this notion of mates looking out for mates: 'in a
SANFL club it's much more social, it's a gathering for business people, local
people, family, mates. You look out for each other'.

Within this category of 'keeping safe', a small number of respondents
mentioned self-imposed rules to limit their consumption of alcohol. These
included no drinking during play, drinking one beer per quarter, no drinking after
half time and a set time to start drinking. Such strategies are illustrative of the
notion of lay knowledge introduced earlier. Here, an understanding of their own
alcohol consumption provides the drinkers concerned with a stock of knowledge
through which to make particular decisions about when, what, how and how much
to drink.

The main strategy for keeping safe, however, was avoiding driving. Many
respondents described how they would arrange alternative ways of getting home
if they were planning on drinking: 'I wouldn't drive or I would work out a way to
[the oval] by public transport. I would get home, depending on how late it finished,
by public transport or by cab' (39-year-old female fan of eastern suburbs club).
Similarly, a 51-year-old make fan of the northern suburbs club notes that:

Forget about the car altogether. Leave it home and catch buses, taxis, whatever.
I always feel responsible when I'm in a group. If there's another guy who says
"look I'll drive" and I know he's going to have a beer or two himself, I'll try and
talk him into sharing a cab or bus with us.

More specifically, the use of a designated driver was commonplace. Terry, a fan
of the eastern suburbs club describes the distribution of driving within the group
of friends with whom he goes to the football: 'we take it in turns. Everyone is
pretty sensible about it. Sometimes the boys in the back [seat] can get loud, but
we share it about'. Similarly, Carole, a fan of the southern suburbs club describes
the potentially tragic consequences of not having a designated driver: 'it's just
what you do. You take it in turns. We've been doing it for years, the four of us.
Sometimes it's a pain, like if the ground's a fair way away, but beats losing your
license or killing a little kid'.

Others spoke of a 'default' designated driver, who's personal circumstances
such as pregnancy, taking medication or particular lifestyle decisions, relegated
them to the role of designated driver, as Phil, a fan of the eastern suburb club

describes: 'Johnno's got one of those troop carriers so he picks us all up in that. He's training for a marathon, dopey bastard, so he's happy not to drink'.

From such accounts, keeping safe was of paramount concern for the drinkers, and they had implemented a number of personal strategies to ensure the wellbeing of their drinking party. Overwhelmingly, it was these tactics, rather than the club-instigated strategies that fans adopted in order to keep themselves – and others – safe.

Minimising the damage
The second theme, 'minimising the damage', described the strategies that drinkers implemented in recognition of the fact that they would, knowingly, be consuming excessive amounts of alcohol over a sustained period. These included eating a substantial meal prior to drinking, spacing drinks with non-alcoholic beverages, and pacing drinking over the course of an afternoon and evening.

The consumption of a meal with a high fat and calorie content was regarded by many as imperative to minimise the effects of inebriation. Martin, a 28-year-old fan of the northern suburbs club, describes his pre-game strategy of '[making] sure I eat enough to soak it all up'. On a 'day on the piss', he tries to 'have a decent big feed. If I know I'm going to have a big session I like to have something in my guts for the beer to float in'.

In addition to lining the stomach, study participants recounted using 'spacers' as a strategy around responsible drinking, as one 28-year-old male fan of the northern suburbs club notes: 'I have some water or a couple of soft drinks. Just pace yourself out if you're making a session of it'. Similarly, Rachel, a 47-year-old female fan of the western suburbs club describes that 'I might drink a few water chasers, if I know we're going to kick on for a while'. Others spoke of rehydrating following an extended session of drinking:

> It doesn't matter how blind I am, I always go home and drink two litres of water. I learnt as a young man that dehydration is probably the main cause of headaches. I always believed in that, so I always drink lots of water when I get home (36-year-old male fan of western suburbs club).

In such comments we see how the respondent's lay knowledge informs his health behaviours. His cumulative knowledge of the after-effects of drinking, informs the decisions he makes about minimising the health effects of sustained drinking.

Taking charge
The third analytical theme, 'taking charge', encompassed strategies in which respondents proactively dealt with another's drinking by letting them know they'd had too much to drink, attempting to slow or stop their drinking, confiscating car keys or money, or distracting them from drinking.

Brigid, a 40-year-old fan of the northern suburbs club describes how she intervenes in what she perceives to be another's dangerous drinking:

I just have a word in their ear and ask them if there's a problem or why they are hoofing them down as much. They might tell me to go and jump in the lake but I will see what the story is and see if I can plant the seed for them to stop.

Paul, a 59-year-old fan of the western suburbs club, recounts a similar tactic: 'I have a relative who tends to over drink. He never gets objectionable, but he's loud and on some occasions I'll say, "Don't you reckon you've had enough? How about slowing it down a bit?"'

When taking charge, several fans described situations in which they would confiscate money or car keys: 'I've taken their car keys a couple of times over the years. Most of the time with your mates, you trust each other. If one says something and the other one backs it up, that sort of calms it down a bit' (Peter, 61-year-old fan of western suburbs club).

In other interventions, interviewees described physically removing a drinker from the bar so as to stop or slow their alcohol consumption. Lee, a 61-year-old fan of the northern suburbs club recounts the following incident:

[We had to] push him out the door to go and watch the game. We got him out of the bar and we had to do it so it didn't get nasty. It was an automatic thing. You know "This bloke's in trouble, we'd better get him out of here" and we just did it. I went outside and starting yelling at the umpires and he started yelling at them and then he forgot all about the bar. Fortunately it worked out. I didn't like the way he was heading. I thought he was heading for trouble and he was a good guy too, but a menace when he'd had a few. One of those you know.

Elsewhere, respondents reported substituting alcoholic beverages for non-alcoholic ones if a person's drinking was becoming cause for concern:

There was a lady who used to drink quite a lot and whenever I could see that she was getting a bit unsafe we would substitute her drinks. Sometimes she'd be clutching the banister so it was a bit of concern. People would switch her drinks … she'd get a bit narky if we took her drink away, so we swapped them over (Amy, 33-year-old fan of eastern suburbs club).

Such comments are interesting, for they highlight the tensions and ambiguities that are evident in these particular strategies for making sense of harm, risk and responsibility. As is the case with keeping safe and minimising damage, the strategies implemented in order to take charge recognise the cumulative body of lay knowledge and expertise that respondents could draw upon to minimise the consequences of drinking and promote more responsible alcohol consumption. In other words, while it is tempting to cast all alcohol consumption in the context of sporting clubs as being risky or reckless, lay knowledge and lay strategies for keeping safe are routinely drawn upon to minimise the potential for harm from some of the behaviours and practices associated with high levels of alcohol consumption.

Such observations, in which sporting clubs are called on to function, in effect, as prevention workers to monitor and reduce alcohol intake among their patrons, alongside efforts to reduce alcohol intake (or to drink sensibly) generated from the bottom up among drinkers themselves, echo the Danish research of Elmeland and Kolind (2012) into the competing discourses of the official public alcohol prevention discourse and an everyday discourse of alcohol use observed among young people and their parents at parties organised for the young people by their parents. As was the case in relation to everyday strategies of keeping safe and formal interventions in sports-associated drinking, the Danish authors found that the public alcohol prevention strategy had a 'general and abstract focus on the health of the population and on the other hand, an everyday practice oriented approach embedded in pragmatic and harm reducing initiatives' (Elmeland and Kolind, 2012: 178). Analytically, these may appear to be contradictory discourses, yet are interwoven in everyday practice with relatively little difficulty.

Resistance and Regulation

The emergence of lay knowledge running either in conjunction with or counter to official discourses and formal strategies and interventions also alerts us to the creative space of resistance and the ways in which consumers re-imagine, re-work and re-interpret the resources attached to health promotion and similar campaigns. While ideas of resistance have their antecedents in notions of youthful rebellion that are found in earlier writings on subcultures (Hall and Jefferson, 1976), the symbolic (and actual) reclaiming of many of the artefacts produced in and through media and popular culture have been similarly re-appropriated in the context of sport-related drinking, and the culture change initiatives aimed at minimising the damage of drinking to excess.

To provide an example, one of the initiatives introduced across sporting grounds in Australia is to only serve beer, wine and soft drinks in plastic cups. The rationale here is that glassware or aluminium cans can be used as weapons or projected as missiles, whereas soft plastic cannot. What observational research at sporting events is discovering however, is that the plastic cups can be stacked inside each other, the 'empties' that are accumulated over a day or evening of drinking coming to represent a marker of drinking prowess (see Figure 6.1). Here the 'beer worms' or 'beer snakes' as they are variously referred to represent a symbolic display of hegemonic drinking through the re-working of a particular initiative designed to reduce the harms associated with sport-related drinking.

While this is a point to which I'll return in Chapter 8, the analytical note to underscore here is that policy makers and practitioners can fail to recognise the limits of policy, and the unintended consequences of well-meaning initiatives. As we saw in relation to the informal and lay strategies that are adopted by drinkers, grassroots initiatives often sit outside 'official' policy responses, and may or may not be in line with formal or government approaches. As examples such as 'the

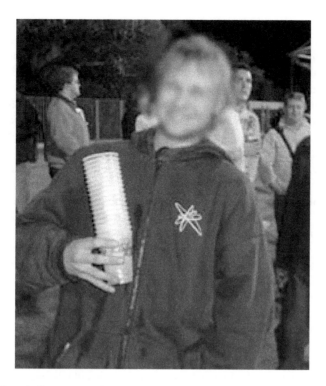

Figure 6.1   A 'beer worm'
Source: Photograph author's own.

beer worm' show, finding ways of changing harmful patterns of intoxication and drunken behaviour can be slow and met with creative resistance.

As with resistance more broadly, this is especially the case among young drinkers, particularly for the adherence to national guidelines for the 'safe' consumption of alcohol. Writing in an Australian context, Roche, et al. (2007) note that young people are less likely to be compliant with alcohol guidelines than older age groups and those aged between 18 and 24 drink at the highest levels of all age groups. Qualitative research among young drinkers aged 20–24 in Victoria, Australia, similarly suggest that their understanding and application of the National Health and Medical Research Council guidelines is low, with many of the young people in the study not seeing themselves as being the subject audience to whom the safe drinking guidelines were aimed at (Harrison, et al., 2008: 8).

Indeed, much of the logic of policy-making ascribes a particular rationality to the 'problem groups' for whom policies, strategies and government guidelines are developed in response to. Policy on 'binge drinking', particularly by young people, is a case in point here. Harrison, et al.'s study of young people's perceptions of the Australian guidelines for 'low-risk' drinking point to some of the reasons for this varied success, arguing that such strategies [of behaviour change] seek 'to engineer in young people forms of personhood that are characterised by similar understandings of the risks they face, and the choices that they should make in relation to their consumption of alcohol in a different way' (2011: 483). While the drinking habits of the young people in the Harrison, et al. (2011) study were well in excess of the recommended guidelines – indeed, participants couldn't think of anyone who drinks within the safe drinking limits – the drinkers nonetheless saw themselves as engaging in 'controlled drunkenness' rather than in behaviour that was particularly risky or harmful; that warranted behaviour change of any kind. As Lindsay notes, 'non-compliance with alcohol guidelines is socially patterned, particularly by age' (2012: 48).

In much the same way, the Grog Squad mentioned at several points already throughout the book clearly engage in drinking that would be regarded as 'binge drinking' under Australian government guidelines, yet they do not regard their drinking as being anything but reasonable. It's simply what they do. Here, context is everything. Although the Groggies drink in a way that is problematic in terms of the amount consumed in a single sitting, it is far from reckless; a notion that underscores the policy debate more generally. For the Grog Squad, drinking is purposeful. It is planned and pre-mediated, bound by group norms and expectations of behaviour and self-control and that are tightly enforced. In other words, a new kind of rationality; one that takes the sociality of drinking seriously is needed for effective policy in the context of sport-related drinking.

Some explanations for non-compliance with the healthy living guidelines have been offered by sociologists and public health researchers. Lupton (1995: 122) has argued that resistance to health promotion advice can occur for a range of reasons including frustration, resentment, pleasure, or even an unconscious imperative to take up alternative subject positions. Thus, resistance to the responsible alcohol messages might constitute anything from 'direct rebellion to simply adhering to the local habitus' (Gjernes, 2010: 474).

Hunt and Evans point to the intransigent paradigm differences between epidemiological research, which 'portrays youthful drug use as particularly dangerous, and young people as especially vulnerable and in need of protection'(2008: 333), and a cultural studies approach which starts from the position that young people are 'active and creative negotiators of the relationship between structure and agency'. Wyn (2009: 9) has argued that promoting the wellbeing of young people is a complex task replete with contradictions that 'invite a consideration of the context of young people's lives, and of the need to connect with their priorities and perspectives in the development of programs intended to help them live well'. Hunt and Evans (2008: 345) have pointed out in relation to drug users that ' … public health messages that fail to acknowledge the enjoyable and beneficial aspects of ecstasy [read alcohol] use will be viewed with doubt and suspicion by many young users'. What remains to be seen is whether such challenges are beyond the neoliberal governmentalities that set themselves the task of managing young people's orientations and dispositions to the use and consumption of alcohol with the aim of promoting young people's health and wellbeing.

Conclusion

This chapter had two key objectives: i) to document the tension between sporting clubs being complicit in encouraging drinking yet compelled to keep their members safe; and ii) to reflect on the contribution that lay knowledge can make to rethinking drinking in the context of culture change. Certainly, 'forward looking' clubs understand that it is in their long-term self-interest to control the use of alcohol, particularly by underage drinkers, where there is a tension between responsible, illegal drinking, for uncontrolled drinking 'contradicts the club's "core business", risks members' health and harms the community through offensive behaviour, violence and drunk driving' (Duff and Munro, 2007: 1992). As I have argued in this chapter however, much of the success in controlling the use of alcohol comes, not from club adopted or enforced initiatives necessarily, but often from the drinkers themselves. This focus on the role of lay strategies in informing health and related behaviours makes an important contribution to how we understand health promotion and policy initiatives in relation to harmful drinking in sport and other contexts.

Such a focus on the drinking practices of sporting fans and the importance of lay strategies in informing health behaviours in relation to alcohol consumption, makes a three-fold contribution to debates about challenging the culture of drinking in sport and the effectiveness of particular forms of health promotion. The data presented in the section on lay knowledge raises important questions as to how clubs could or should regulate and set policy on the relationships between sport and alcohol, given that drinking to get drunk is very often a deliberate, pre-mediated choice in this context. As described here, drinkers were aware of the consequences of inebriation, yet they persisted. This problematic nexus of knowledge and choice is recognised by Lhussier and Carr who write that 'only if we know enough about healthy lifestyles can we act responsibly towards them' (2008: 303).

Such empowerment discourses also allow us to 'stop thinking' and act irresponsibly with regards to our lifestyle choices. That is, we know enough to decide what to take on board and what to ignore. The strategies deployed by the drinkers in this research suggest they know enough about keeping safe to counter the harmful effects of what they know is going to be a day of irresponsible, health damaging behaviour. As I have argued throughout the book, treating the fun and pleasure of peer drinking as a legitimate source of meaning is crucial for understanding some of the difficulties with ensuring effective policy compliance. The hedonism of drinking presents club officials, governing bodies and policy makers with a dilemma, for it clashes with other expectations of citizens, including notions of responsibility, reasonableness and self-control, where negotiating the tensions and contradictions inherent in the pleasure of drinking raises a whole set of questions for research, policy and practice (Coveney and Brunton, 2003; Measham and Brain, 2005; Harrison, et al., 2011).

Second, acknowledging the pleasure associated with acts of determined drunkenness has particular consequences for the presentation and interpretation of accounts of drinking (in sport or elsewhere), and these are not easily reconciled in the broader context of the governance and regulation of alcohol consumption that is situated in a policy discourse of harm minimisation and harm reduction. As Hutton notes 'harm reduction has long struggled with interventions in drinking because of the tensions between its pleasures and the damage caused' (2012). Drinking with your mates can be enormously good fun, and accounts of calculated hedonism and determined drunkenness do not always sit comfortably alongside debates about harm minimisation, risk and regulation that are part of a broader policy agenda on 'binge drinking', particularly among young people, and raise critical questions such as how to write about the enjoyment and pleasure of the sociality of drinking, sport-related or otherwise, without celebrating or valorising it? That has certainly not been my intention here.

Third, notions and understandings of pleasure raise equally difficult questions of definition and measurement. 'Having fun' is a crucial narrative in the promotional culture and practices of the alcohol industry, yet where, and how, do we draw the line about what constitutes the fun of drinking? Or, indeed, what constitutes responsible drinking? Is staying sober the only form of responsibility, or is planning for getting plastered, to return to the premise of the AMO, equally responsible, despite individuals clearly intending to drink to excess from the outset? Following on from this, how do we develop policy and legislation that can regulate mateship, friendship, belonging and peer norms, for these are essentially the cultural drivers of sessional or heavy episodic drinking in sport or anywhere else.

Such questions, I suggest, raise further ones about the boundaries of acceptability, and pleasure. Getting 'shit-faced' – to use the Australian vernacular – isn't every one's idea of fun, but it is for others, and therein lies the rub. Boundaries, definitions and assumptions of what constitutes fun, reasonableness, control or recklessness – the fundamental debates that are at work here – speak to a broader discussion about the 'disconnect' between healthy living guidelines and lived or embodied practice. Here, the debate involves more than simply alcohol. Food, exercise, time spent in the sun, or in front of the television, are all subject to guidelines for 'healthy' or recommended limits that are often, substantially at odds with how much food, exercise, sunshine or screen time people actually consume. As Lindsay notes 'health eating and healthy living guidelines invite us to manage our bodies in an ideal, individualised world where lifestyle change is a straightforward matter of putting knowledge into practice' (2011: 475), yet, as the actions of groups like the Grog Squad described in earlier chapters suggest, groups and individuals may draw on different forms of knowledge – such as knowing what feels good – in their disregard of 'low risk drinking' guidelines.

As I have suggested here, the 'disconnect' between policy and behaviour ignores the social contexts within which the behaviour occurs, and the very real and legitimate meanings that are attached to health damaging behaviours such as the sport-associated drinking described in the book. In many cases, alcohol consumption clearly exceeded the national guidelines for recommended drinking in a manner that suggested a deliberate disregard for health promotion messages, in doing so, contradicting the expectations of rationality, reasonableness and risk awareness that underpin the policy drivers of governmentality and citizenship. While my interest here is in sport-related drinking, such issues are of relevance to other contexts that bring people together to drink (or consume other drugs) in ways that are 'objectively' health damaging. Building on this, the following chapter takes a different approach to culture change in the context of sport-related drinking.

Chapter 7

Some Paradoxes and Potentials for Recovery and Prevention

This chapter:
- explores the relationship between sports-based interventions and alcohol use and misuse;
- reviews the growing trend for sport to be used in health and welfare programmes that encourage young (usually male) people to make better choices in relation to alcohol use;
- considers the contradictory discourses that surround the use of 'sport' in health, welfare, recovery and treatment programmes.

Introduction

A key feature of government policy in most Western neoliberal democracies is the use of sport programmes or sports-based interventions as a vehicle for social change in relation to social problems, including those pertaining to alcohol misuse. Here, sport is promoted as either a diversion from a range of health damaging, anti-social or criminal behaviours that are associated with dangerous alcohol consumption, or is used as an intervention that can provide opportunities for treatment and rehabilitation. In both cases, marginalised and vulnerable population groups, most often young people in urban areas who are considered to be at risk of offending, have been the focus of these kind of programmes and initiatives. It is the paradoxical and, at times contradictory, nature of the relationship between sports-based interventions and alcohol use and misuse among young people, in particular, but not exclusively, that informs this chapter.

The chapter reports on research that examines and questions the effectiveness of sports-based interventions in relation to problematic alcohol consumption among young people, and the ways in which the 'sport-alcohol nexus' (Palmer, 2011) is increasingly being regarded as a space for treatment, desistance and prevention work by a number of practitioners keen to explore the benefits of sport for the 'positive development' of urban youth. The particular biases that are implicit in such assumptions of 'benefit' or 'positive development' are explored in the ensuing pages.

Following Spandler and McKeown (2012), the chapter examines the 'paradoxical spaces' of sports-based interventions and the two competing and, at times, contradictory discourses that run through accounts of alcohol-related sports-based initiatives and strategies. The first is the 'mythopoeic' narrative (Coalter, 2007), in which sports (usually football and basketball) are promoted – largely uncritically – as an opportunity for prevention, rehabilitation and recovery from many of the social problems associated with alcohol misuse. The second is the 'counter-mythopoeic' narrative, in which the potential for sports-based interventions to *reproduce* rather than redress structural inequalities is highlighted as an unintended consequence of what Giulianotti (2004) has referred to elsewhere as the work of 'sports evangelists'. Here, questions of efficacy, evidence and the effectiveness of these sports-based interventions are raised in relation to alcohol use and misuse.

The chapter unfolds as follows. It begins with a brief review of the growing trend for sport to be used in health and welfare programmes that encourage young (usually male) people to make better choices in relation to alcohol use, and its associated social costs and consequences. The Positive Futures programme and the Homeless World Cup provide the research backdrop here. To consider the utility of those schemes which are aimed at supporting people through their *recovery* from alcohol and drug misuse, the chapter focuses, empirically, on research conducted by Sarah Landale (2012; Landale and Roderick, 2013) on the Second Chance programme in the United Kingdom. From here, the 'paradoxical spaces' within which such schemes and personal narratives sit is interrogated. Here, the chapter turns to something of a critique of the contradictory discourses that surround the use of 'sport' in health, welfare, recovery and treatment programmes before posing some questions and recommendations that may help shape future research and practice-based programmes, particularly, but not exclusively, in terms of youth development and alcohol use.

Sport, Alcohol, Health and Welfare

The ways in which sport has been used as a means through which to tackle a broad range of social issues and problems have been well-documented. Much of the literature comes out of Western neoliberal democracies, including the United Kingdom (Blackshaw and Crabbe, 2004; Coalter, 2007; 2013a; Magee and Jeans, 2011; Kelly, 2010; 2012), the Netherlands (Spaaj, 2009; 2013; Haudenyhuyse, Theebom and Nols, 2102) and Australia (Morris, Sallybanks and Willis, 2003; Palmer, 2009). Much of the focus of these sports-based initiatives is on crime prevention and/or crime reduction, and many of the programmes share similarities in their structure and intent, as well as the population groups (usually young males) who are targeted through such interventions.

While the focus of this chapter is on sports-based interventions as they relate to alcohol use and misuse among young people, this broader context provides a useful framework within which to locate such health and welfare programmes, for the premises on which they are based are, in many ways, very similar. Borrowing from the Respect Task Force established by the former Labour government in the United Kingdom to 'provide constructive and purposive activities [that can] encourage and enable children and young people to contribute to their communities and help divert them from anti-social behaviour' (Respect Task Force, 2006: 10), such sentiments are echoed in much of the discourse, rhetoric and practice that surrounds sports-based interventions as they relate particularly to alcohol consumption by young people in the UK and elsewhere.

Indeed, themes of self-transformation and personal development, the importance of supportive peer relationships, the provision of safe spaces and alternative activities are common to accounts, evaluations, and indeed critiques of sports-based interventions across the broad terrain of social inclusion and health and welfare. Of particular concern for this chapter, sports-based interventions that are intended to tackle problematic alcohol use by young people or problematic population groups fit broadly within the 'sport-plus' model (Coalter, 2007), in which sport as either a concept or a practice is conceived as a hook or as a way of attracting young people into programmes that are less about sport and more about offering services, information and advice. Here 'free access to sport [is] used as "fly paper" to attract young people, or defined widely and used as a reward and a social context for intensive youth work' (Coalter, 2013b: 599).

Often run in conjunction with other youth services (such as health, employment or vocational training) these programmes address a range of health and welfare issues that may stem from problematic or risky alcohol use (i.e. run ins with the law, unplanned sex or pregnancy, injuries, and so on). In other words, sports-based initiatives are constructed and conceived as the point at which social and individual and wider health problems, as they relate to alcohol misuse, coalesce or come together.

Public health campaigns, for example, have used the involvement of young men in football (soccer) as a way of endorsing the importance of physical activity to healthy living (Robertson, 2003; White and Witty, 2009), as well as using football to engage (young) men who may be marginalised or stigmatised through mental health concerns (Carless and Douglas, 2008). The gendered nature of such initiatives not withstanding (and echoing the book's concern with a masculine bias in approaches to sport and alcohol more broadly), sports-based interventions that relate to endorsing better choices around alcohol use or engaging those who may be marginalised as a result of their alcohol misuse are located firmly within this 'sport-plus' framework.

Prevention

Relative to that available to older populations, considerable provision is made, in most Western neoliberal democracies, for sporting activities for young adults and marginalised youth groups that may help deter them from engaging with alcohol in problematic ways (Crabbe, 2013). The original Positive Futures scheme, for example, is a nation-wide sport and activities-based social inclusion programme, delivered across 91 sites in England and Wales. Aimed at young people aimed between 10 and 19 years of age who are at risk of drug misuse or offending, the programme seeks to offer access to personal development opportunities through sport and physical activities. Here, partnerships are established between sporting and non-sporting agencies (such as the police or training agencies) that use sport and other developmental activities, including a range of lifestyle, educational and employment activities to achieve the intended outcomes of reduced offending and substance misuse among young people.

While developed initially in the United Kingdom, similar schemes bearing the Positive Futures moniker have been rolled out in other parts of the world, including Brazil (Spaaj, 2012) and Australia, where the principles of the scheme have been implemented in remote Indigenous communities such as the Wujal Wujal settlement in the Cape York Peninsula area of far-north Queensland. As is the case elsewhere, this variation of the Positive Futures programme is run in conjunction with the police (in this case the Queensland Police-Citizens Youth Welfare Association), and it aims to reduce the risk of young people coming into contact with formal statutory processes such as the youth justice system, as well as improving young people's participation in society, particularly in education, training and employment through the effective use of creative community partnerships across sports, arts and cultural providers.

Elsewhere, the Choose Life, Choose Sports programme run by the Government of the Republic of Macedonia through the Agency of Youth and Sport adopts a 'social marketing' approach to communicate the harmful impacts of alcohol and drug misuse (and smoking) on young people's health and wellbeing (Dimovski and Paunova, 2012: 229). Employing popular Macedonian athletes such as Indira Kastratovik, Kiril Lazarov and Darko Pancev, these athletes serve as safe drinking champions to promote responsible drinking among young sportsmen and women (Dimovski and Paunova, 2012: 229).[1]

While this is a point to which the chapter will return, the 'plus' benefits of such sport-plus schemes notwithstanding, there is often considerable slippage in the intentions, delivery and audiences for such schemes, with outcomes around crime reduction, social inclusion and substance misuse frequently blurred and taken to be one and the same. Such observations echo similar concerns to those raised in the previous chapter about 'long and thickly populated intervention chains' (Pawson and Tilley, 2004: 5). That is, such schemes, in discourse and practice, can be seen as a one-stop-shop where all manner of social problems can be mitigated, and there is a need to more critically assess the evidence and the effectiveness of targeted schemes against specific outcomes for very particular social problems, in this case alcohol misuse, rather than relying on the global gloss of the mythopoeic narrative.

---

1   Darko Pancev is a football international; Indira Kastratovik and Kiril Lzarov are handball players with the Macedonian national team.

Indeed, Tim Crabbe (2000), who undertook a series of evaluations of the Positive Futures programme, argues for the need to 'de-centre' sport in order to understand which sports work for what subjects, under what conditions. More recently, Crabbe refers to such sports-based interventions as being 'cultural intermediaries' and he identifies the need to consider concepts 'centrally concerned with the intimate dynamics of human relations' and the need 'to mobilise these concepts in a fashion which actively seeks to ... contribute to the design of the community sport project' (Crabbe, 2008: 34–5). In other words, Crabbe argues for a need to obtain 'a deeper understanding of the complexities of participants' interactions and the often contradictory and fluid impact of initiatives' (Crabbe, 2008: 34–5).

As well as sports-based interventions that seek to divert or prevent young people from entering or continuing with problematic relationships to alcohol, sport is slowly, but increasingly, being used as an intervention and an opportunity for *recovery* and *rehabilitation* programmes for many of the social problems associated with alcohol misuse.

Recovery

In contrast to the use of sport as a preventative intervention, sport has played relatively little part in alcohol and drug *treatment* programmes, despite the well-established health benefits of physical exercise (Department of Health, 2010) and the knowledge that many people with alcohol and other drug problems are, and want to be, physically active (Neale, et al., 2007). Indeed, the appeal of sport and exercise can be seen in different ways, and with different levels of intensity, among people dealing with addiction. Studies suggest, for example, that many prisoners engage in organised physical exercise and sport while in prison and some gain related qualifications, but few continue with sporting activities, or use their qualifications, on release because of the problems associated with social exclusion (Meek and Lewis, 2012). While the debates around the often assumed benefits of sport is a point to which I will return, there is, in theory, much that could be gained by supporting people with alcohol and other drug problems to do more exercise through their treatment and recovery journey.

Limited research has examined the contribution that sports programmes may make to young people's recovery from addiction (and again Positive Futures is instructive here – cf. Crabbe, 2000), but to date sport has played little part in *adult* alcohol and drug rehabilitation programmes. Calton Athletic Recovery Group in the United Kingdom is one of the few programmes to use sport as a change agent in an addict's recovery journey, yet despite, this, there remains something of a reluctance to use sport and physical exercise as an alternative or an adjunct to established psychological and pharmacological interventions (Landale and Roderick, 2013).

That said, research on the concept of 'natural recovery' has identified that meaningful activities are a key part of resolving alcohol and drug problems

(Granfield and Cloud, 2001), and it is here that Landale's life-history-based research with adults recovering from alcohol (and other drug) problems and their involvement with a sports-based intervention is particularly insightful. Over a period of 12 months, Landale conducted research with participants (or clients) involved with the Second Chance programme, a community-based drugs intervention programme in the United Kingdom that offers a range of sporting and other activities (such as theatre and debating) to help self-identified 'addicts' to stay clean. Working with adults, as distinct from youth, who are not in education, training or employment, Second Chance adopts the 'sport-plus' model (Coalter, 2007) to draw on the support and resources of a range of non-sporting organisations, including drug and alcohol recovery centres, homeless organisations and remand and probation officers, to facilitate desistance from substance misuse.

Throughout her research, Landale was concerned with examining how participants attached a broad range of social and symbolic meanings to Second Chance over the course of one year in the context of their recovery, and, more particularly, how they situated their engagement with Second Chance within the context of their other routine activities over a 12-month period. Employing a 'life-course approach' that examined the use of informal social controls, transitions and turning points in an addict's journey through recovery, Landale's study explored the meanings that participants attached to Second Chance in the wider context of their everyday lives. Recognising that situational contingencies and routine activities can either tempt people towards or away from addiction (Sampson and Laub, 2005), Landale's research was concerned with the ways in which the stuff of everyday life may help or hinder recovery. As Landale and Roderick note 'overcoming addiction requires some degree of self-change, and for this process to happen, facilitating opportunities are required' (2013: 15).

As was the case with those programmes intended to divert those at risk of substance misuse, schemes such as Second Chance which are aimed at supporting adults through their recovery from drug or alcohol misuse, tend to be far less about the 'sport' and more about the non-sporting or the 'plus' activities that are partnered to such programmes. Writing about Second Chance, Landale and Roderick note that recovery was 'facilitated through a confluence of meaningful routine activities, informal social controls and personal agency, both within and outside of Second Chance' (2013: 1).

Returning to the notion of situational contingencies or 'entire systems of social relationships' (Pawson and Tilley, 2004: 7) as underpinning a broader concern with 'what works' in sports-based interventions, Landale's research alerts us to the importance of locating behaviour change, such as withdrawal, recovery and abstinence within the context of the life-course of an alcoholic or addict. Without this, the contributions that sports-based interventions may (or may not) make in either recovery or prevention are stripped from the individual's life and their worldview. In this respect, life-course criminology can offer, as Williams notes, 'further insight about the significance of transitions to adulthood which can be applied to decisions about drug taking' (2013: 13).

Making Sense of Recovery

In the field of alcohol and drug research, social capital is a key concept employed to explain the resources (financial, material and human) that those recovering from addiction may, to varying degrees, draw upon to facilitate their recovery. Extending this, the concept of 'recovery capital' has much traction, with literature suggesting that recovering addicts who have higher levels of recovery capital were better able to desist than those without (Best and Laudet, 2010). Alongside this, theories of identity and the presentation of self (after the fashion of Erving Goffman, 1959) have emphasised the role of identity (re)construction among addicts as they move into and out of addiction and, following on from this, they ways in which individuals attach meaning to their lives, relative to the changing centrality of drugs in their lives (McKintosh and McKeganey, 2002). There are limitations, however, with both a social capital driven approach and an explanation driven by a recasting, symbolically, of one's identity. Social capital can overstate the structural aspects of what moves people to behave in certain ways, while symbolic approaches to identity (re)construction can place too much emphasis on identity and agency aspects of behavioural change. A life-course theory, by contrast, charts a middle course between the two, integrating elements of structure and agency (Landale, 2012). Certainly, life-course theory, and the transitions and turning points it invariably includes, return us to the 'age-old debate about the significance of structure versus agency and the significance of culture' (Williams, 2013: 14), in which agential decisions about drug-taking (including consuming alcohol) are framed within cultural and structural circumstances or locations.

Life-course Perspectives on Alcohol Use

Life-course criminology, as the term implies, is concerned with studying the development of deviant or criminal behaviour over time from onset, persistence to desistance and the impact of life events upon such behaviour. Landale's (2012; 2013) research sought to pinpoint transitions and turning points in adulthood that may either lure people towards or away from addiction. Implicit in the theory is the methodological necessity of allowing people to speak of their recovery journey, thereby highlighting the important role that personal biographies play in narrating that journey. As detailed in Chapter 5, narratives of addiction, demise and recovery are powerful cultural scripts, yet it is rare that we hear of 'the journey' of recovery in terms of sport-related drinking. In other words, the words of the addict can serve as both a tool of analysis (as discussed in Chapter 5) and a tool in recovery, discussed in this chapter.

Rethinking Drinking and Sport

Landale's research with clients of Second Chance employed a life-course theory of informal social controls similar to that adopted by criminologists Laub and Sampson (2003). Developed from a longitudinal study undertaken in the United States to chart desistance among formerly incarcerated young men in Boston, the life-course theory of informal social controls recognises three mechanisms that can help us to better understand persistence and desistance. These are: (i) 'routine activities'; (ii) 'informal social controls'; and (iii) purposeful 'agency', with the interaction between the three being best described as 'situated choice'. In other words, behaviour – such as persisting or desisting – is the result of both the context in which people with chronic substance misuse problems live (the 'social environment') and their own personal agency.

While Laub and Sampson (2003) describe agency as 'choice', stating that this is as important as routine activities and social controls when examining persistence and desistance across the life-course, they also drew a distinction between choice as agency and rational choice theories, stating: 'choice alone without structures of support, or the offering of support alone absent of a decision to desist, however inchoate, seems destined to fail' (Sampson and Laub, 2005: 43). Specifically, agency was defined as 'choice', but differentiated from rational choice and situated in the social and environmental circumstances within which an individual was located at any given point in time. Thus, choice is determined by a complex and dynamic set of interrelated variables which include a person's past and present experiences (e.g. addiction or homelessness), while at the same time constantly needing to move forward.

The acts of 'doing things', such as routines, habits and practices (Nettleton, et al., 2011), as well as the cognitive processes involved in choosing to desist (Biernacki, 1986), also influence choice, even when an individual cannot easily account for their actions or does not want to (Gadd, 2006). The interaction of routine activities, informal social controls and agency was described as 'situated choice' in which agential processes such as decisions to drink, take drugs or commit crime are linked to situations such as opportunities or social network and larger structural factors such as marriage or full-time employment. Applying the life-course perspective to drug abuse, Hser, et al. (2007) noted that turning points vary; that is, the same event can trigger a change in one person's drug use but not another's, and this will depend on the individual and the context.

While Landale's research focussed on a small number of respondents, it allowed an in-depth examination of their cognitive processes as they attached meaning to Second Chance, in the context of their day-to-day lives in their recovery. From this perspective it was only through in-depth, theoretically selected case studies that are 'sensitive to the latent or unconscious meanings of respondents' narratives, including all the absences, contradictions and avoidances intrinsic to them' (Gadd and Farrall, 2004: 132) that agency could be captured and understood.

Discussing the use of life-course perspective in relation to alcohol and drug abuse and turning points, Groshkova and Best state that 'within a life-course model, there are "windows of opportunity for change" that represent the turning points [out of addiction] in a developmental trajectory. The challenge for science is to identify when and why these occur and what makes the changes sustainable' (2011: 37). For Landale and her study participants, Second Chance represented a 'window of opportunity for change' (Groshkova and Best, 2011: 11) within which one participant may be experiencing a 'turning point', while the other was not. For Landale, this turning point was conceptualised as an identity change, and was dependent upon the respondent's other routine activities, social networks and personal agency (choice) both within and outside Second Chance (Landale, 2012; Landale and Roderick, 2013). Thus for desistance to happen, respondents needed other networks of support in addition to Second Chance; that is, they needed the 'plus' aspects of the sport-plus model. In recognising this, the life-course perspective thus offers a useful approach to explain and understand problems related to alcohol and other drugs, and how these interrelate with social systems which structure people's lives (Groshkova and Best, 2011).

As research with these practice-based programmes (i.e. Positive Futures or Second Chance) suggest, teasing out the impact, reach and intended audience is very often a complex, circuitous pathway, with linear links to cause and effect far from clear cut. This then returns us to questions of efficacy, evidence and the effectiveness, and the potential for sports-based interventions to *reproduce* rather than redress structural inequalities in programmes aimed at either deterrence or desistance from alcohol use and misuse.

Having sketched the broad terrain within which sport is implicated in both the prevention and recovery from alcohol-related harms, the chapter turns now to theorising the 'paradoxical spaces' within which such schemes sit. It considers the mythopoeic and counter-mythopoeic narratives that help account for the contradictions and tensions in the sport-alcohol nexus outlined in the chapter so far.

The Mythopoeic Narrative

In essence, 'mythopoeic concepts' are those whose 'demarcation criteria are not specific, but are based on popular and idealistic ideas that are produced largely outside of sociological analysis' (Coalter, 2013a), and the strength of such myths lies in their 'ability to evoke vague and generalised images' (Glasner, 1977: 1).

The mythopoeic narrative that surrounds sports-based interventions argues that they work because it is assumed that there is something inherently good and noble about sport. Crabbe, for example, notes that 'the notion of the "power of sport" to do social good [and] belief in the wider benefits of sport has rarely been so strongly advocated' (2008: 22). Indeed, as evidenced in examples like Positive Futures or Second Chance, this notion of the 'power of sport' to tackle a whole raft of social problems and to 'improve' the lives of the individuals and communities in which they live has been readily adopted by governments, health practitioners and community development workers, among others. As Coalter notes, 'the most consistent rationales underpinning public investment in sport (usually assumed to be competitive team games) have been based on the supposed moral component of sport and its ability to teach 'lessons for life', to contribute to 'character building' (e.g. honesty, integrity, trustworthiness), to contribute to the development of self-discipline and deferred gratification and positive moral reasoning (Coalter, 2013b: 597).

This rationale was accelerated and reinforced in the UK by the then 'new' Labour government's policies to address the multi-faceted problem of 'social exclusion', a major component of which was crime and high-crime environment (Coalter, et al., 2000; Collins, et al., 1999; Social Exclusion Unit, 1998). This led to a proliferation of sports-based programmes aimed at addressing issues of social exclusion and aimed at at-risk youth.

In the United Kingdom, the social inclusion agenda within which programmes like Positive Futures or Second Chance operate is based on assumptions about the 'potential contributions [of sport] to areas such as social and economic regeneration, crime reduction, health improvement and educational achievement' (Coalter, 2007: 1). Similarly, in Australia, the social inclusion agenda is embraced in relation to marginal and vulnerable groups such as Indigenous peoples (Cunningham and Benaforti, 2005) or refugee and migrant communities (Palmer, 2009; Spaaj, 2013), particularly in terms of achieving health and wellbeing outcomes that are indirectly related to sport. My own work, for example, details the ways in which participation in a community-based soccer programme for young Muslim refugee teenage girls enables the participants to develop networks and social capital within their neighbourhood and community more broadly (Palmer, 2009). In the case of Indigenous youth in remote Australian communities, targeting alcohol and other substance misuse (petrol or glue sniffing) has been a part of a broader (some argue punitive) approach to engaging those who may be marginalised as a result of their alcohol misuse, isolation and limited opportunities for employment or education (Brady, 1992).

As such examples suggest, these government agendas – and the initiatives that sit within them – are largely based on uncritical assumptions of inevitably positive outcomes. In other words, sport 'works' simply because it is sport. Indeed, the mythopoeic status of sport is particularly acute when it comes to youth development. As Coakley writes 'there is widespread belief that sport participation inevitably contributes to youth development because sport's assumed essential goodness and purity is passed on to those who partake in it' (2011: 306).

In terms of initiatives intended for dealing with problems related to alcohol misuse among young people, the majority are premised uncritically on the assumption that sport 'does good' for young people at risk of psychological or physical harm as it: 'structures their lives around mainstream values and goals; removes them from the streets and consigns them to adult-controlled environments; teaches them self-control, obedience to authority and conformity to rules and provides them with positive adult role models' (Coakley, 2011: 308).

While these claims are also made for sports-based interventions more broadly, the narrative resonates with those initiatives intended to achieve outcomes relating to reducing the risk of drug and alcohol misuse or facilitating recovery for those experiencing addiction. Such claims, as Coakley notes, are based on the assumption that involvement in sports-based interventions produces what he calls the 'car wash' effect – that is, it 'cleanses character and washes away personal defects so that young people become acceptable to those in mainstream society' (2011: 308). In the case of schemes targeting Indigenous youth in Australia, New Zealand or Canada, there are added assumptions here about white, middle-class normativity that may 'restrict certain individual actions whilst enabling others' (Magee and Jeanes, 2011: 6).

However, there is a tension here that begins to alert us to the 'paradoxical spaces' of sports-based initiatives as they relate to young people and drug and alcohol misuse; that is, the *unintended* consequences of encouraging young people into sport as a way of discouraging their alcohol use, and associated social problems. Crabbe puts it succinctly:

> The fact that the same emotions of excitement, euphoria, celebration, tension and fear are being used does not suddenly result in drugs no longer being seen as "fun" or worthwhile. Indeed where the competitive nature of sport results in people not "making the grade" ... they may subsequently become disillusioned and alienated by sport to the degree they may seek solace in the more "reliable" effects of drug use (2000: 390).

The Counter-mythopoeic Narrative

Not surprisingly, the counter-mythopoeic narrative raises such unintended consequences as critical concerns for the individuals and communities that the initiatives are meant to help, as well as for the rigour of academic scholarship, evidence-based policy making and, indeed, the veracity of the initiatives themselves.

The counter-mythopoeic narrative arises from a critique of sports-based interventions on several levels. It is, for example, acknowledged that evidence as to the effectiveness of sports-based interventions relating to deterrence or desistance from alcohol misuse is limited – either because robust and comparable monitoring and evaluation has not been undertaken consistently (Coalter, 2007) or there are major and often inherent methodological difficulties in measuring the impact of programmes (Nichols, 2007; Nichols and Crow, 2004). Secondly, as Coalter, (2013b) notes 'sport is a collective noun that hides more than it reveals. Such diversity and the major limitations that it places on easy generalisations were emphasised by the President's Council on Physical Fitness and Sports (see Figure 7.1).

From the President's Council on Physical Fitness and Sports:

For several reasons, broad generalizations about 'sports' are unlikely to be helpful. For one, the rule structures of the various sports promote different types of social interaction. The developmental stimuli provided by a boxing match are likely to differ from those of a golf tournament. In addition, each sport tends to have its own subculture and implicit moral norms. The culture of rugby is quite different from that of competitive swimming. ... Even within a single sport area and developmental level, individual sport teams are different because each team develops its own unique moral microculture through the influence of particular coaches, athletes, fans, parents, and programs. Moreover, even within a single team, participants' own appraisals of the experience may vary substantially (2006: 4).

Figure 7.1   From the President's Council on Physical Fitness and Sports

While part of the counter-mythopoeic narrative and its implicit critique of sport-plus programmes emerges out of the evaluative research which suggests that sports programmes on their own are most unlikely to cure social problems, including that of addiction (Landale and Roderick, 2013), the concern here is more with the social and structural inequalities that sport-plus programmes, as they relate to drug and alcohol misuse, have the potential to reproduce. For example, examining sports-based interventions for young socially excluded people, Kelly (2011) found that despite the benefits (such as enabling people who would otherwise not have been able to access sporting facilities), projects often did not meet the aims they predicated themselves on, such as tackling social exclusion. There was also little impact made by the projects in addressing the socio-structural foundations from which young people became excluded in the first place.

Borrowing from the literature on sport and international development more broadly, the implications of the counter-mythopoeic narrative are significant for more fully understanding the paradoxical spaces of sports-based interventions as they relate to drug and alcohol misuse, prevention and rehabilitation. Indeed, the stinging critique of sport and international development has resonance for more local interventions around substance misuse. The essence of the argument advanced by scholars in the field is that many of the assumption upon which particular interventions are premised are reproduced in uncritical forms, and are 'used by well-meaning people and organizations from wealthy nations to justify the creation of sports programs for populations that lack participation opportunities and face challenges caused by poverty, war, natural disasters, or oppression' (Coakley, 2011: 307). While Coakley writes about tensions that emerge, largely, from relationships between the Global North and Global South or, more crudely, the developed and developing worlds, his sentiments strike a chord with sports-based interventions as they relate to young people and alcohol misuse, particularly the intentions of 'well-meaning' workers to effect change among individuals and communities who neither want nor see the need to change behaviours.

Indeed, sociologists such as Darnell (2010), Hartman and Kwauk (2011) and Coalter (2007; 2013b) have been especially critical of the ways in which personal testimonials from those delivering sport-plus schemes have become the 'evidence' that is used to argue for the success of the scheme. In particular, it is the ways in which the outcomes of such programmes have been framed in terms of the personal development and transformation of the young *individuals* who take part in such schemes with little recognition of either the need for structural change at a community or societal level, or the potential that their presence in the community may do more harm than good that, in this context, forms the basis for the counter-mythopoeic narrative.

While this is a complex argument to unravel, there are two inter-related issues that underpin the critique as it relates to young people and alcohol use and misuse: i) an emphasis on the presumed empowering and transformative properties of sport, while downplaying or failing to consider the wider social and structural concerns that may have given rise to the problem the initiative seeks to address and; ii) in doing so, reproducing rather than redressing the wider structural inequalities that are experienced by the target individual and communities.

To provide just a couple of indicative examples, Spandler and McKeown note that 'football initiatives represent both the potential to tackle the thorny issue of a relative lack of engagement of men in constructive reflection on their health and well-being' (2012: 388). However, they also raise the peril of uncritically 'reproducing damaging constructions of gender and inequalities that are not unconnected to men's health outcomes and social problems' (2012: 388). Writing about disadvantaged youth in the Netherlands, Spaaj similarly questions the 'uses of sport-based intervention programs as a vehicle for social mobility and contends that 'in many cases the program fails to break through the system of social reproduction' (2009: 262). Research into the ways in which the Homeless World Cup may help combat social exclusion among homeless people has been conducted (Sherry, 2010; Magee and Jeanes, 2011; Ravenhill, 2008) which also questions the 'extent to which the relationships that players develop by participating in the tournament may actually entrench players in the homeless culture rather that provide routes out of homelessness' (Magee and Jeanes, 2011: 8). While these sports-based interventions do not specifically target alcohol misuse, substance abuse remains a consistent undercurrent in such programmes, with many participants homeless, isolated or disadvantaged as a consequence, in part, of their drug and alcohol use. As Magee and Jeanes note of participants in the Homeless World Cup, 'all smoked and were heavy alcohol drinkers with two admitting to alcoholism and the majority acknowledging a history of substance abuse' (2011: 9).

In relation to sport-plus programmes, particularly, but not exclusively as they relate to young people at risk of or recovering from drug and alcohol misuse, there is a need to consider the extent to which sports-based interventions in fact challenge or reproduce unequal social relationships. It is argued that participation in sports-based initiatives does little more than further stigmatise at-risk groups and the broader assumptions that are brought to bear on particular population groups, such as young people, particularly young people who drink to excess. That is, by taking part in such schemes, participants are already singled out as 'problematic' in one way or another, and taking part in the programme only serves to reinforce their problematic status.

While the reproduction of stigmatising stereotypes and structural inequalities may be the unintended consequences of sport-plus programmes and the mythopoeic narrative, it is worth reflecting on some of the contributing factors that give rise to the rhetoric and practice of sports evangelists. Critics such as Coakley (2011) or Coalter (2007; 2013a; 2013b) have consistently argued that one of the issues with sports-based interventions, as they relate in this case to substance misuse, is a critical lack of rigorous evidence that can substantiate – empirically – the feel-good presumptions that the programme has achieved its outcomes or, concomitantly, that can document the failures and limitations that need to be redressed in future iterations of a programme. As Coakley writes:

> Over the past century, the claims of sports evangelists have informed and justified sport-related program and funding decisions at local and national levels, despite a general lack of research support … They are accepted to such an extent that even when progams fail repeatedly, neither are their critical evaluations of the culture and organization of sports or the contexts in which sports are played and given meaning nor are there critical examinations of the dual assumption that sport is essentially good and that its goodness is automatically experienced by those who partake in it (2011: 309).

Coakley's contention that there is little convincing empirical evidence of impact, outcome or effectiveness is particularly compelling in the context of monitoring outcomes around substance misuse and young people. In light of arguments about the need to better understand context, structure and agency, positivist evaluations that focus solely on outcomes such as a reduction in alcohol consumption are fairly meaningless. While there is no question that a reduction in heavy alcohol use can lead to better physical and mental health outcomes, there is a need also to look at the wider social forces that may also enable better choices around safer alcohol use, along with any assumed causal links between participation in a scheme and reduction in alcohol use, better treatment outcomes or a reduction in alcohol-related crime, violence and social disorder.

Where to From Here?

While the 'mythopoeic' (Coalter, 2007) nature of sport and its ability to adequately address complex social problems has been problematised in relation to community interventions and outreach work, sports-based alcohol intervention programmes continue to command considerable policy attention and government and private sector funding. Although the counter-mythopoeic narrative can be quite damming, I am not suggesting we do away with such schemes; rather that scholars and practitioners remain alert to the potential of such programmes to reproduce rather than redress structural inequalities and to further stigmatise the very individuals and communities that such schemes are meant to support.

In light of this, it seems that adopting a middle-ground approach may be a pragmatic way forward. That is, many sports-based interventions that relate to drug and alcohol misuse and recovery do trade on the capital stock of sport and it is important to acknowledge that, for many individuals and programmes, sport is an effective hook. At the same time, we need to recognise that sport alone cannot achieve outcomes around drug and alcohol diversion or desistance, but successful partnerships between sports delivery and non-sporting organisations may well contribute to better choices and outcomes around health and wellbeing. Following on from this, it is imperative to recognise that by targeting groups deemed to be 'at risk' of substance misuse (or criminal activity or social disorder), we run the risk of singling out such individuals as 'problem people' and further reproducing the stigma and structural inequalities in which they are already implicated and embedded.

Given the 'paradoxical spaces' of sports-based interventions and the two competing and, at times, contradictory discourses that run through accounts of alcohol-related sports-based initiatives and strategies, what might be some of the questions for future research and the conditions within which such schemes may more effectively operate?

- In terms of research methods and data collection, there is a need for more ethnographically informed research that can better understand how young people learn about and come to know and understand the factors that negatively affect their lives and how they make choices around these things.
- There is also a pressing need for researchers to better understand contexts of drug and alcohol use. Both the mythopoeic and counter-mythopoeic narratives suggest that, as researchers and practitioners, we know or assume a great deal about the 'power' of sport, but we know far less about culture and context as it relates to young people and their drug and alcohol use.
- At the same time, we need to provide evidence for the contextual factors that may serve as pre-requisites for positive outcomes around alcohol diversion and desistance. We know that participation in sport is more likely to occur when it takes place in settings where young people are physically safe, personally valued, morally and economically supported, personally and politically empowered, and hopeful about the future (Hellsion, 2003; Walsh, 2008).
- Questions of efficacy, evidence and the effectiveness of sports-based interventions in relation to alcohol use and misuse remain fundamentally linked to questions of design and delivery. Coalter (2007) highlights the

often poorly conceptualised and articulated outcomes of many sport and social development programmes, arguing the need for a more logical approach to both project inception and evaluation. Programmes that address diversion and desistance from drug and alcohol misuse are equally implicated here.

- despite the benefits which exercise programmes potentially offer to those recovering from drug and alcohol misuse, mainstream funding has tended to favour pharmacological and psychological interventions which have focused on reducing the harms associated with alcohol and drug misuse. Correspondingly there is little research, and even less prospective research, into how sport and exercise may help people resolve alcohol and other drug use issues and help maintain sobriety. Much more is needed in this space.

Conclusion

This chapter has been concerned with the 'paradoxical spaces' (Spandler and McKeown, 2012) of sports-based interventions and the two competing and, at times, contradictory discourses that run through accounts of alcohol-related sports based initiatives and strategies. The chapter has argued that the power of the rhetoric that surrounds these initiatives often obscures damaging and stigmatising practices and assumptions, and opens up the potential for these initiatives to reproduce rather than redress many of the structural inequalities that have given rise to the initiatives in the first place. I chose, intentionally, not to provide an analysis of any one programme, rather to suggest that the paradoxical spaces and contradictory discourses that surround alcohol-related sports-based interventions as either preventative or rehabilitative options, are indicative of Pawson and Tilley's contention that 'intervention chains are long and thickly populated. Interventions carry not one, but several mechanisms of action' (2004: 5).

Drawing on the mythopoeic and counter-mythopoeic narratives, I suggest that the most effective models for sports-based interventions as they relate, in this case, to alcohol misuse and recovery are those that adopt the middle ground. That is, those that to some extent embrace the feel good aspects of the mythopoeic narrative as well as recognising the need for critical reflection on intentions, assumptions, processes, programmes and outcomes that are embedded within the counter-mythopoeic narrative. In other words, sports-based initiatives are *both* mythopoeic and counter-mythopoeic in their discursive and practical constructions. They can both address alcohol-related harms among people *and* reproduce some of the structural inequities and social fractures the initiatives are intended to address. Therein lies the paradox. As I address in the following chapter, negotiating the paradox and related contradictions in the sport-alcohol nexus as it relates to policy development, implementation and uptake is especially difficult, particularly when overlaid with the, at times, competing interests of marketing, sponsorship and the promotional culture of sports-associated drinking.

Chapter 8
Policy and Sponsorship

This chapter:
- considers the relationships between sponsorship and policy-making in the context of sport and alcohol;
- suggest new directions for wider debates and concerns about regulation, responsibility, access, affordability, risk, harm and pleasure.

Introduction

So far, the chapters in the book have been principally concerned with expanding the research agenda around the sociality and social contexts of sport-related drinking. They have questioned the over-riding emphasis on hegemonic masculinity as a theoretical perspective for explaining and interpreting many of the behaviours associated with sport-related drinking, and they have introduced new conceptual possibilities for understanding sport-related drinking through frameworks such as calculated hedonism, determined drunkenness, symbolic capital and governmentality, as well as offering new empirical examples including non-drinkers, female drinkers and drinking that takes place among alternative sporting communities – such as roller derby and Ultimate Frisbee – that run against the grain of traditional orthodoxies of sport-related drinking.

This emphasis on widening the theoretical and empirical understandings of sport and alcohol also raises some important questions for an emergent policy agenda, particularly, but not exclusively in terms of health and social issues. As I suggest in this chapter, an expanded sociological perspective on sport-related drinking that engages with cultural practices, social meanings and lived experiences can also help inform policy and practice issues and debates in ways that policy makers (and sociologists) are increasingly recognising. As Measham notes [there is a need] for 'greater understanding of why and how people drink in order to design culturally appropriate, evidence-based harm minimisation strategies that can be communicated in credible and effective ways' (2006: 258).

While much of the policy attention is directed towards harm minimisation as it relates to the health of drinkers at an individual and population or public health level, alcohol policy is also bound up in a legal framework of licensing, regulation and restrictions that dictates where, when, who, how and how much an individual can drink. At the same time, sport is widely accused of being a servant to the aggressive promotional culture which seeks to sell alcohol in particular ways to particular sections of the community, using major events and prominent or celebrity athletes to do so.

This intersection of health policy and the promotional culture of the sport-alcohol nexus means that the two are often held in tension with one another. That is, policy and practice aimed at harm minimisation and regulation sometimes make uneasy bed fellows for marketing and sponsorship, with many of the practices intended to promote the consumption of alcohol leading to the often held view that sport is awash with alcohol sponsorship; that is, a handmaiden to the alcohol industry. In other words, policy as it relates to harm reduction in the context of sport (and more broadly) brings together bodies and organisations who are involved in an intricate interplay of contested, sometimes complementary, interests that are often about emergent forms of governmentality that are translocal and cross-national, as well as transnational in their reach and rule.

The contradictory nature of sport-related drinking, as both a source of pleasure, identity and sociality, and one of considerable costs and consequences for health and wellbeing presents a number of issues and challenges for health and public policy and it is not in the least bit surprising that the two present something of a discursive disjuncture. The seemingly contrasting discourses of (responsible) pleasure and one of regulation and restraint offer a useful way of framing some of the key developments in public policy as it relates to government and industry-led initiatives and directives, and those that relate to health promotion and wellbeing more broadly. Using the sociological lens that informs much of the book, this chapter is principally concerned to understand the context and the mechanisms through which policy is created, regulated, reproduced and resisted by individuals and communities in the context of sport, health and welfare.

The chapter unfolds as follows. It begins with a discussion of the marketing and sponsorship of alcohol in sport. It then turns to some of the implications for policy, particularly, but not exclusively, in terms of health and social policy. The mutually reinforcing relationships between sport and alcohol and the role the two play in producing key social relationships raise a number of questions and suggest new directions for wider debates and concerns about regulation, responsibility, access, affordability, risk, harm and pleasure, which are reviewed and critiqued in this penultimate chapter.

Alcohol Marketing and Sponsorship of Sport

There is little doubt that there are strong financial links between alcohol and sport or that the alcohol industry is heavily invested in the marketing and sponsorship of sport and sporting events. As Wenner and Jackson write, 'in the United States alone, of the approximately $1 billion spent on alcohol advertising, 60% of it supports sports programming' (2009: viii). Somewhat more pithily, Jacobsen observes in an Australian context that 'whether it is the Melbourne Cup, motor racing, cricket, or any code of football, when the winners step onto the podium they will probably thank an alcohol company for sponsoring them' (2003: n.p).

Sport and Alcohol Sponsorship

Around the globe, manufacturers of alcoholic drinks, particularly beer, are major sponsors of sporting teams and events. In the United Kingdom alone, breweries are heavily present in their sponsorship of both football (soccer) and rugby. The Carling brewery, for example, sponsored a national football league along with a number of football and rugby clubs. Celebrating '36 years of football and Tennents', the Scottish brewer sponsored both the Celtic and Rangers teams (in something of a national monopoly on the game). Elsewhere, the American-based Budweiser is one of the official sponsors of the FIFA World Cup (managing to fight off 'ambush marketing' in 2006 from the unofficial Dutch-based Bavaria Brewery), and the global reach of Budweiser vis-à-vis football's World Cup was discussed previously in Chapter 4. The Greek brewer Athinaiki Zithopiia (Athenian Brewery S.A.) was one of the sponsors of the Athens 2004 Olympic Games, while in Australia, Bundaberg Rum and VB (Victoria Bitter beer) are two of the sponsors of the national (men's) cricket team. The perceived disconnect of using an arguably unhealthy product (beer) to promote an arguably healthy set of practices (sport) is not lost. As Wenner notes 'how is it that alcohol consumption in the face of athleticism is not portrayed as a cultural irony? How has this come about? How is it that the sports fan feels at ease in judging athletic prowess with a beer can in hand?'(1991: 391–2).

As noted in Chapter 4, however, the religious beliefs of some athletes present a challenge to this normative expectation of alcohol sponsorship in sport. Fawad Ahmed, a Muslim player with the Australian cricket team, for example, refuses to wear the official team uniform because it features the logo of the beer sponsor VB, an action that followed the precedent of Hashim Amla, who took the same stance with an alcohol sponsor of South Africa's cricket team.

Nonetheless, the close association between alcohol (usually beer) and sport is made possible by coherent social constructions of sport that have great currency globally. As Wenner and Jackson note 'the selling of sport and the selling of beer have been blended ... Beer seeks a ride on the logic of sport and sport rides on beer' (2009: 11). The relative stability of particular sports myths and dominant orthodoxies certainly assists in this, in particular, the recurrent narrative theme that sport and drinking are assumed to be two key sites where notions of masculinity are played out.

As I noted in Chapter 2, the consumption of alcohol and the successful enactment of drinking (and drunkenness) is widely regarded in Western, neoliberal and democratic societies as being among the quintessential or archetypical practices through which particular forms of masculine identity can be explored, enacted and embodied. Certainly, the alcohol industry recognises the male market – that 'breweries have historically spent the bulk of their advertising dollars in sports programming where desirable 18–49-year-old men congregate speaks to their allegiance to the manhood formula' (Wenner and Jackson, 2009: 14). Moreover, because alcohol is a consumable – it is drunk and it is gone, 'it is an ideal focus for continual advertising to trigger repeat sales' (Chrzan, 2012: 111).

While traditionally, beer companies have been involved with the sponsorship of sporting events such as the football or rugby World Cups where the logic of globally televised sport dominates the programming space, increasingly we are seeing commodity culture as it relates to the sport-alcohol marketing nexus now being played out on many media platforms. Traditional media such as newspapers and magazines are still popular, yet alcohol companies are entering the space of new media, where we see sport-programmed websites, blogs and video games, among others, promoting alcohol brands, extending the user-generated content already seen on YouTube and social networking sites such as Facebook, Twitter, Myspace and the like. In the United States, for example, the brewing giant Anheuser-Busch launched, in 2009, Bud.TV in an attempt to expand its marketing reach beyond a television audience alone. Tens of millions of dollars were spent by the brewer on building, in effect, an entertainment network for its Budweiser beer brand, with content being created by writers and performers from the comedy stable of the television programme *Saturday Night Live*.

Relatedly, new media and social media in particular also feature heavily in terms of the pervasiveness of content about drinking within user-generated material on social networking sites (McCreanor, et al., 2013; Brown and Griggs, 2012). 'Selfies' and stories of inebriation frequently memorialise a user's 'big night out' across social networking sites yet, at the same time, social media and web-based platforms are being used to promote (and document one's progress) through Australian and New Zealand health promotion initiatives such as such as 'Hello Sunday Morning' http//hellosundaymorning.com.au), FebFast (http//febfast.org.nz) and Dry July (http//www.dryjuly.com). While these innovations signal the potential of health promotion approaches to using multimedia channels such as blogging, social networking sites and YouTube, these social marketing campaigns nonetheless face the challenge of trying to 'de-normalise alcohol consumption in a deregulated environment that is saturated with alcohol marketing determined to achieve the opposite effect' (McCreanor, et al., 2013: 116).

The increasing globalisation of sport, alcohol sales and market penetration has particular implications for the commercial imperatives of the sport-alcohol nexus. According to Collins and Vamplew 'the increasingly global nature of sports brands … makes them even more attractive to an industry which itself is consolidating across national boundaries into 'super-breweries' [such as Belgium's Interbrew], making marketing and advertising campaigns simpler and cheaper' (2002: 123–4). Reflecting on the announcement that Heineken would be the Official Beer Supplier and a Worldwide Partner for the Rugby World Cup in England in 2015, the Chief Commercial Officer for Heineken, Alexis Nasard, announced in her press conference that:

As the world's most international premium beer brand, we are delighted again to be an integral part of the world's premier rugby tournament for 2015. Rugby World Cup is the world's third largest sporting event, with a truly global reach. It is a perfect match for Heineken, and allows us to be a genuine part of our consumers' conversation in a consistent but surprising way. It also gives us the continued opportunity to extend our messaging and execution around *Enjoy Heineken Responsibly*, the brand's global responsible drinking programme (Reuters, 2012).

This close association between alcohol sponsorship and sporting events has given rise to a number of scholarly treatments and interpretations, many of which are usefully summarised in Wenner and Jackson's (2009) edited collection *Sport, Beer, and Gender in Promotional Culture: Explorations of a Holy Trinity.* Attentive to the inequities that are embedded in sport, Horne and Whannel (2009) argue for the importance of social class in considering the connections between sponsorship, sport and alcohol. Drawing on 'a degree of reflexive auto-ethnography', and a 'search of advertising archives and other documentary sources', Horne and Whannel (2009: 56), suggest that social class, in the UK at least, provides a means of identifying differential, gendered relationships to sport as well as to types of alcohol as well: 'social class and gender continue to shape culturally transmitted conceptions of both appropriate types of alcohol consumption and drinking cultural practices and sports participation and involvement' (2009: 73). In other words, there is a mutually reinforcing relationship between sport and alcohol in 'fashioning promotional strategies and shaping culture of consumption' (Wenner and Jacskon, 2009: vii). Institutional practices and marketing strategies establish and legitimise particular contexts for alcohol consumption, such as sporting events, which see alcohol brought to the market through sport, leading to the observation that 'anyone involved in sport, whether as a player or as a fan, will almost inevitably be exposed to a strong message that alcohol and sport are inextricably linked' (Jones, Phillipson and Lynch, 2006: n.p).

Mega-events and the Sport-Alcohol-Advertising Nexus

As I began to suggest in Chapter 4, alcohol sponsorship is an intrinsic part of staging global sporting mega-events, with major alcohol companies being named partners of several events that attract global media audiences in the order of several million people. As noted previously, the beer company Heineken is the official beer supplier and a worldwide partner for the Rugby World Cup in England in 2015, while Budweiser is a worldwide partner and sponsor of football's World Cup. As I noted in Chapter 4 however, hosting the 2022 FIFA World Cup in Qatar; an Islamic country where the 'use of alcohol is especially troubling for Muslims, who may be deeply offended if they are in the vicinity of alcohol' (Dun, 2014: 186) poses some critical questions for this dimension of the sport-alcohol nexus.

In terms of the Rugby World Cup, naming Heineken as the official beer supplier and a worldwide partner extends Heineken's long-standing association with rugby's showcase event. Heineken first partnered with Rugby World Cup in 1995, yet the new agreement allows Heineken to maintain access to a package of worldwide rights, including designations in promotional tie-ins and digital content rights across a host of social media channels. While this is a point to which I'll return, the analytical note here is that the globally mediated nature of these events has given rise to a particularly influential group of cultural intermediaries who are increasingly involved in setting the policy agenda and the mechanisms of communication across a broad range of social and commercial issues.

As we saw in Chapter 4, the host nation of the 2014 football World Cup experienced the iron first of FIFA who coerced the Brazilian government, despite the Health Minister, Alexandre Padilha, and other members of Congress calling for the ban to be maintained, to change a law that has prohibited the sale of alcohol in Brazilian sports stadiums since 2003 in order to protect the commercial rights of Budweiser, one of its World Cup sponsors. As I have argued elsewhere (Palmer, 2013c) there is no doubt that sporting bodies such as the Fédération International de Football Association or the International Olympic Committee (IOC) are powerful organisations who enjoy wealth, celebrity, status and global influence on a scale with few rivals.

International alcohol sponsorship reforms
Despite the interventions of cultural brokers in influencing national policy as it relates to alcohol consumption at sporting events, in several countries, policy and legislation have been introduced that seek to regulate the advertising and promotion of alcohol (less so, its consumption) at sporting events. While the discourse of the overt promotion of alcohol may seem at odds with a discourse of regulation and restraint, these discursive fissures are symptomatic of a highly contested policy arena in which competing interests and agendas jostle with one another.

When debates around the regulation of alcohol appear on the policy agenda, the example of France's *Loi Évin* (or Evin Law) is commonly cited. Implemented in 1991 to protect against risks and harm to public health, *Loi Évin* bans alcohol advertising on television or in cinemas and prohibits alcohol sponsorship of cultural and sport events. Thus, despite alcohol companies being closely tied to sporting mega-events such as the football or rugby World Cups, the annually occurring Tour de France cycle race remains entirely free from alcohol promotions and sponsorship. In addition, under *Loi Évin,* all advertising must include the health message: '*l'abus d'alcool est dangereux pour la santé*' (alcohol abuse is dangerous to health).

To return to the rugby World Cup, when France hosted the event in 2007, Heineken was also a Worldwide Partner and the official beer of the tournament, contravening *Loi Évin*. Infringements to the Law during the 2007 Rugby World Cup were highlighted by a formal complaint lodged from ANPAA (the *Association Nationale en Alcoologie et Addictologie)* in response to Heineken advertising banners being circulated to café and bar owners, along with Heineken print advertisements portraying imagery affiliated with a rugby game including an oval-shaped beer glass depicting a rugby ball. The court ordered Heineken to either remove the advertisements linked to the 2007 Rugby World Cup within 48 hours or accept a fine of €5000 per violation. Arguably, while *Loi Évin* remains, for many, a blueprint for regulatory practices against alcohol advertising and sponsorship, it is important to note that *Loi Évin* does not restrict the *sale* of alcohol at sports events in France, raising issues for those concerned with the health and social effects of excessive single session or 'binge' drinking.

Alcohol Policy: Regulation and Restriction

The competing discourses surrounding alcohol – and sport – have seen sport-related drinking occupy a persistent presence on the policy agenda. It remains a 'wicked' problem that cuts across sports, agencies, governments, authorities and nationalities. It is an on-going policy problem for sporting organisations, departments and agencies worldwide.

Broadly speaking, policy as it relates to alcohol (in sport or elsewhere) can be categorised as policy that is concerned with availability and affordability and policy that is concerned with minimising the harmful impacts of dangerous levels of alcohol consumption to individuals and communities. Clearly, the distinction is a blunt one made for reasons of analytical simplicity. In reality, there is overlap between the two policy domains, with policy seeking to regulate the sale of alcohol also being concerned with public health. Following Babor, et al., I argue that 'public health relies on policy and regulation as the most effective ways of reducing the negative impacts of alcohol; through decreasing population-level consumption and encouraging harm-reduction in high-risk drinking contexts' (2010: 17).

Liberalisation and Regulation

Alcohol availability, affordability and promotion have increased markedly in the last three decades as a result of liberalised central and/or state government alcohol policies. In most Western, neoliberal democratic countries, the liberalisation of national and/or state alcohol policies has had a major impact on the availability of alcohol, yet not necessarily in terms of *reducing* its availability. In New Zealand, for example, national government policy based on a free-market ideology has seen the number of licensed premises increase from 6,000 to over 14,000 (including supermarkets and grocery stores) over a period of six years. The minimum purchase age has also been reduced from 20 to 18 years and the sale of alcohol is available 24 hours a day, seven days a week (Casswell and Maxwell, 2005). By contrast, the sale and distribution of alcohol in Norway is regulated by national policy through a state-owned liquor monopoly as well as taxation in order to limit the sale and distribution of alcohol to liquor stores only (Beccaria and Sande, 2003: 106).

Alongside policies that seek to restrict the availability and affordability of alcohol, laws that punish driving while under the influence of alcohol have been similarly effective in reducing some of the harms of alcohol consumption (i.e. road toll) globally. While these changes are not in, and of, themselves about alcohol policy in the context of sport, they nonetheless provide an important backdrop against which sport-related drinking can be considered. As Maclennan, Kypri, Langley and Room note, there is considerable evidence to suggest that 'in the general population, policies restricting alcohol availability and promotion are the most effective tools for the prevention of hazardous drinking and associated harm' (2012: 45).

Indeed, in their systematic review of research on the efficacy of strategies for reducing alcohol-related harm, Babor, et al. (2003) consistently found that measures such as the use of price, taxation and availability were recognised as the most effective evidence-based approaches to reducing alcohol-related harm. Globally, effective policies include a legal drinking or purchase age of 20 years or higher, higher alcohol taxes, lower blood-alcohol concentration driving limits, restrictions on the number and density of alcohol outlets in communities, limiting the hours and days of the sale of alcohol and the strict enforcement of liquor laws regarding sales to underage and intoxicated persons (Esenbach-Stangl and Thom, 2009; Barbor, et al., 2010).

As well as policy seeking to limit the availability and affordability of alcohol, a raft of policy initiatives and health promotion innovations have been developed that foreground issues of safety among drinkers. Key here are concerns with the physical safety of the people using licensed premises, not with broader alcohol-related public health issues. Again, while these are not in and of themselves about sport-related drinking they nonetheless provide an important backdrop to initiatives such as the Alcohol Management Operation or the Good Sports programme discussed in Chapter 6. With a nod to some of the debates about the night-time economy, alcohol-fuelled violence, drinking curfews and drinking cordons that were introduced in early 2014 in some of Australia's most notorious 'party zones' (such as Sydney's King Cross or Brisbane's Fortitude Valley), the introduction of these kind of initiatives strike a delicate balancing act between maintaining order and control and not stifling the very conditions of the night-time economy that attract many people in the first place (Hobbs, et al., 2003).

What is important here is that many of these safety-based policies or schemes are premised on arguments of 'drunkenness' and intoxication', yet as indicated in Chapter 1, there is little consensus as to what these terms mean and how they might be defined. Levi and Valverde explain some of the difficulty of defining such a slippery concept as intoxication:

> The legal entity of intoxication has an inherent tendency to undermine and indeed deconstruct, the opposition between opinion and fact evidence.

Eyewitnesses can and do give evidence that they saw Mr X consume three beers or, more commonly, that Mr X was swaying while walking, had bloodshot eyes or whatever. But the addition of a few such observations so as to produce the aggregate, somewhat diffuse, category of intoxication is a tricky epistemic operation (2001: 835).

Despite such fears, concerns with 'intoxication' remain the cornerstone of a range of highly restrictive policies that limit individual choice and responsibility as to where, when, how, why and what they might drink. In the context of sport-related tourism, for example, such restrictive policies demonstrate Brain's (2009) 'evident tension' between consumer excess and the need for moderation and restraint. While some of the challenges that the construction and representation of sport-tourism destinations as 'party central' locations has been noted in previous chapters, the imposition of these restrictions that dictates where, when, who, how and how much an individual can drink raise questions of balance for the promotional dimensions of events such as the Ashes Test, and travel for the Barmy Army or rugby 'Sevens' events and the four-yearly World Cup (Gee, Jackson, and Sam, 2014).[1]

This balancing act returns us to some of the debates about risk that I introduced in Chapter 2. As noted then, there is a fundamental tension in writing about sport and alcohol and, indeed, alcohol consumption more broadly, namely that between the regulation or mitigation of risk and ideas of pleasure and enjoyment. Of concern here is the way in which the management of the 'risks' of drinking to excess has entered the policy arena for, as Pike notes 'once a situation is defined as risky, it is then also political, since governments and individuals are required to attend to it' (2007: 311). This construction of risk is an inherently social act; as Douglas (1992) notes, it is through the subtle valuing and imposition of particular futures – the prioritising of certain actors' values at the expense of others – that risk becomes a political tool. In the case of sport-related drinking, and drinking more broadly, we see a culture of risk meet with a culture of caution, where 'one person's risk may constitute another person's pleasure' (Mythen, 2004: 182) or where 'good' risk meets 'bad' risk. It is in this space where, I suggest, most health and social policy is conceptualised and constructed.

Health Policy and Sport-related Drinking

Despite the commercial imperative to link the promotional culture of alcohol with the promotional architecture of sporting events, the increasing levels of alcohol consumption in most western countries, and the associated health, social and economic harms are key public health concerns that can neither be denied or

---

1   Rugby Sevens or 'seven-a-side' is a variation of rugby union where instead of the usual 15, teams are made up of seven players. Rugby Sevens is now recognised as an Olympic sport and will make its debut at the 2016 Summer Olympics in Rio.

ignored, and it is with this acknowledgement that alcohol policy is conceived and implemented.[2]

As Babor, et al. (2003) note, alcohol policy broadly refers to those measures aimed at minimising the harms that result to both individuals and society as a result of alcohol use. Indeed, globally, national policies and strategies contain a wide range of prevention, treatment and harm reduction responses to the problems of intoxication and unacceptable drinking behaviours. As I outline here, harm reduction covers a range of possible interventions, the common feature of which is merely that they do not aim at abstinence. In this respect, harm minimisation may refer to health practitioners working with individual drinkers to help them to manage their alcohol consumption with greater insight; to strategies and interventions designed to modify public drinking environments (such as the changes to the Australia's drinking party zones, which have recast the spatial dimensions of the night time economy); or to adapting aspects of public policy so as to encourage moderation through taxation or the control of opening hours of licensed venues. As Measham notes:

> [Harm minimisation] aims to reduce the harm to the individual and society from the manufacture, marketing and consumption of legal or illicit drugs through the application of measures that priorities decreasing the risks and severity of adverse consequences from current use over the reduction or elimination of use per se. In relation to alcohol, consumption can result in harm from drinking itself (such as health outcomes) and when combined with another activity (such as driving or operating machinery) (2006: 259).

Broadly speaking, harm minimisation strategies take a threefold approach to prevention and intervention: i) universal prevention that is aimed at a whole population; ii) selective interventions that are aimed at high-risk groups and; iii) systemic changes to the physical, drinking environments. I look now at these in terms of sport-related drinking.

Universal Prevention Aimed at a Whole Population

The prevalent belief in many 'wet cultures' such as Australia or the United Kingdom is that alcohol consumption is intrinsic, taken for granted, 'banalised' and expected, and this has profoundly shaped public health discourse and practice towards harm minimisation. Operating from the standpoint that alcohol use will continue in these and other countries, efforts are thus directed towards reducing

---

2 The Alcohol's Burden of Disease in Australia 2010 Report, for example, suggested that injuries (including motor vehicle crashes) accounted for 36 per cent of alcohol-related deaths among men during the previous year, followed by cancer (25 per cent) and digestive diseases (16 per cent). For women, cardiovascular disease was the leading cause of alcohol-related deaths (34 per cent) followed by cancers (31 per cent) and injuries (12 per cent).

any harm associated with drinking rather than advocating abstinence (Hutton, 2012; Rumbold and Hamilton, 1998).

Several sport-related social marketing campaigns therefore adopt this logic to form partnerships between a sporting club or organisation and a related company or government department so as to encourage widespread behavioural or attitudinal change towards some of the consequences of excessive alcohol consumption. For example, the Transport Accident Commission (TAC) in Victoria, Australia, has been involved with the sponsorship of several sports, notably Formula 1 Grand Prix and Australian Rules football, using the high profile media coverage of both sports to promote awareness of road safety, particularly drink driving, speeding and fatigue. In various TAC campaigns over the years, football players have been the public face of the 'Wipe Off 5' campaign to promote driver safety; they have been involved in initiatives to discourage speeding among young male drivers and they have featured in campaigns aimed at reducing drink driving.

Invariably, however, tensions can emerge, given the 'mass-media cycle of celebration, transgression, punishment and redemption' (Turner, 2004: 106) within which much of global sport and its sponsorship operate. In the mid-2000s, several players from two of the TAC sponsored clubs were caught speeding or drink driving (in one case, five players from a single club) compromising the lucrative sponsorship deals between their clubs and TAC. In a reversal of what Schaaf (2005) has described as 'lightning in a bottle'; the moment when something beneficial or influential happens that can be associated with the product, the involvement of these players in serious traffic infringements resulted in the termination of the club's sponsorship deal with TAC. Yet, curiously it also brought about the kind of wholesale 'shaming' of players that the several of the TAC television campaigns featured as their dominant narrative device.

Such universal prevention programmes, then, that are aimed at promoting particular kinds of behaviour at a population level seek to encourage moderation by educating 'the public' about the harms of their or other's behaviour, so as to reduce the associated health and social costs, without constraining individual liberty. Indeed, as noted in Chapter 2, a key focus of the 'new public health' (Baum, 2008) is that public health initiatives such as alcohol harm minimisation campaigns are a form of governance 'at a distance' (Rose and Miller, 1992: 184–6) through which the good conduct of citizens is promoted through forms of governmentality and risk watching.

Once again, the concept of risk comes through, for so much of policy is formulated around populations 'at risk' – children at risk of obesity, risk factors for chronic health conditions, drinkers at risk, for example, and the concept has become central to how social relations are organised and governed through social and public policy. Here, Foucault's concept of 'governmentality' helps frame the logic of risk-based policy making. For Foucault, governmentality refers to the 'art of government' in which government has 'as its purpose not the act of government itself, but the welfare of the population, the improvement of its condition, the increase of its wealth, longevity, health etc.' (1991: 100).

Selective Interventions Aimed at High-risk Groups

While the governmentality of universal prevention programmes tends to operate at a population level, most harm-minimisation strategies, in sport or elsewhere, tend to be aimed at particular 'high-risk' groups such as young women. As Measham notes 'the traditional focus of alcohol education and prevention has been the reduction in demand for and use of alcohol through public health programs targeted at "at-risk" groups. Despite mixed evidence to the effectiveness of these strategies, they remain a key priority' (2006: 260).

To provide just two examples, a multi-media campaign from the Canadian province of Saskatchewan aimed at young adults aged 19–29 raises awareness of the risks and consequences associated with excessive drinking so as to promote the responsible use of alcohol, and modify alcohol drinking habits in the province. Similarly, the 'Don't turn a night out into a nightmare' campaign from Australia depicts a series of scenes involving 15–25-year-olds in binge drinking gone wrong. One advertisement depicts a teenage girl getting drunk at a house party and eventually having sex on the lawn while being filmed by laughing party-goers. It finishes with a reminder that one in two teenagers will do something they regret while drunk. Another shows a girl downing several drinks and cutting herself after falling on a glass table.

In terms of sport-related drinking, selective interventions aimed at high-risk groups similarly target young people. As outlined in Chapter 6, structured interventions such as the Good Sports programme or the AMO were established with the expressed intent of 'regulating the use of alcohol within sporting clubs, producing a permanent change in drinking customs' (Duff and Munro, 2007: 1991) and responding to the more immediate risks and dangers of excessive drinking by high-risk groups. Many sporting clubs are doing quite extraordinary work, particularly with under-age drinkers, and in rural and regional communities, as the AMO attests to, and the considerable challenges that they face in bringing about meaningful and sustained cultural change is acknowledged, given that ways of changing harmful patterns of intoxication and drunken behaviour can be slow and met with creative resistance, as outlined in Chapter 6.

In terms of health – and related – policy, the premise that underpins these and similar club and community-based interventions is that sporting clubs can operate as important sites for health promotion (Kelly, King, et al., 2014). Part of a broader settings-based approach to health education in which healthcare and messages about healthy (and at-risk) behaviours can be communicated in a variety of non-traditional settings (such as general practitioners offering check-ups in the pub or nursing professionals offering sexual health checks at county fairs), such strategies are ultimately aimed at developing a range of alcohol management strategies that can transform local drinking cultures in community-based sporting clubs, particularly among those groups identified to be at-risk.

The paradox, however, of using sporting clubs as health promotion settings was alluded to in Chapter 6, and this tension between the role of sport in promoting healthy behaviours, and sporting clubs as a site for unregulated and dangerous drinking, *as well* as the use of sports-based interventions to prevent a range of anti-social activities or to assist with treatment and rehabilitation from alcohol-related harms is clearly a contradictory or paradoxical space, to return to one of the ideas from the previous chapter, with shifting agendas and multiple narratives at work that are not always or easily reconciled.

Systemic Changes to the Physical and Drinking Environments

To turn to the third prong of harm minimisation strategies, systemic changes to the physical and drinking environments tend to be less the domain of sports-based interventions and more the domain of community-focussed strategies. By way of illustration, we see, particularly in Northern Europe and the United Kingdom, prevention programmes that seek to change the community structure or the environment in which alcohol consumption occurs. In other words, alongside 'official' responses, there are many attempts by voluntary and lay organisations to set up initiatives to respond to problem drinking behaviours in their local areas.

As I discussed earlier in the chapter, both alcohol availability and its promotion have increased markedly in the last three decades as a result of liberalised central and/or state government alcohol policies. As such, many communities are relying on the people within or on local governments to manage alcohol problems. A key example here is the UK Community Alcohol Prevention Programme (UKCAPP) and its community prevention approach championed by Holder (2000; 2004).

The Holder approach
To put this in context, In the United Kingdom, the UK Community Alcohol Prevention Programme (UKCAPP) seeks to change the communities' structure or the environments in which alcohol consumption occurs. Using the cities of Glasgow, Cardiff and Birmingham as pilot sites, the 'Holder approach' takes its point of departure a distinction between 'traditional' and 'environmental' concepts of communities. Holder highlighted a long history of 'traditional' alcohol harm reduction interventions in communities (media campaigns, alcoholism recovery services, and school educational interventions), which he argued miscast 'communities and reduced interventions to programs within a community rather than broader policy-based practices across a society. With traditional understandings of community conceiving it as a 'catchment area for a specific target population with interventions developed to affect that group ... as long as the existing social, economic and cultural structures remain unchanged, the potential effectiveness of these interventions in reducing alcohol problems is limited' (Mistral, Vellerman, Templeton and Mastache, 2006: 280).

Unlike the previous two models of harm reduction, the 'Holder approach' does not require the identification of at-risk drinkers or groups, nor their active co-operation. Instead, efforts are directed towards local policy makers in positions to influence the environment. As Mistral, et al. note 'local alcohol policy can be used to alter the community's social, economic or physical structures and put in place processes and priorities to reduce alcohol problems' (2206: 280). In such a model or approach, policy and policy makers (rather than the drinkers) are the target for action, where strategies such as 'prioritising alcohol-related problematic behaviour by the police, controlling location and density of alcohol outlets or ensuring server training for all licensed premises' (Mistral, et al., 2006: 280) are key parts of the policy equation. As outlined in Chapter 6, these kind of 'intervention chains are long and thickly populated' (Pawson and Tilley, 2004: 5), where it is often difficult to separate out which aspects of the intervention contribute to its effectiveness.

Nonetheless, notions of harm minimisation have much currency in policy debates among Western neoliberal democracies, where the term (and rhetoric) covers a range of possible interventions, from health practitioners working with individual drinkers to help them to manage their alcohol consumption through to strategies and interventions designed to modify public drinking environments. All, however, bring into play a certain tension around the need for government or policy intervention into drinking behaviours, and, in doing so, raise a series of questions as to the extent we want to what governments to control drinking behaviour, to educate us on responsible drinking, or to protect us from alcohol-related violence, among other things?

Implicit too, is the idea of risk. In terms of policy making, it is crucial that those who promote and regulate health, welfare and safety in sport, including alcohol consumption, understand how people think about and respond to risk; that is, who appreciate the tension between subjective and objective experiences of risk. While risk is clearly a contested social construct, we live in an era that is increasingly risk conscious, and policy discourse and decision-making, in relation to both sport and alcohol reflects this.

A Sociology of Sport and Alcohol Policy

I started the chapter with the assertion that an expanded sociological perspective on sport-related drinking that engages with cultural practices, social meanings and lived experiences can also help inform policy and practice issues and debates. This then, invites the question as to how a sociologist would interpret the contested terrain of alcohol *policy*, rather than alcohol consumption addressed in previous chapters, as it relates to sport.

I have argued elsewhere (Palmer, 2013c) that policy is not a 'neutral' process but one that is always socially constructed; the product of considerable cultural work on the part of a whole range of individuals and organisations. In other words, policy is essentially a 'thing' that is created by some and implemented by others, and it is imperative that we understand who is involved, how, where, when and why in the development and delivery of policy instruments as they relate to sport and alcohol or, indeed, sport and social policy more broadly. This raises two questions that are explored below: who does the constructing of policy and what are the consequences (real or imagined) of that construction?

Cultural Intermediaries and Policy-making

From the chapter so far, it should be fairly evident that it is increasingly rare (and difficult) for governments to take governing decisions about drinking without including the corporate (advertising and sponsorship) and voluntary and non-government sectors (harm minimisation, care and welfare) in the process. Forming a 'policy network' of actors aligned by mutual interest and resource dependence, it is the assumptions and frameworks which underpin the processes through which this takes place that this chapter has been largely concerned with.

As I've written about elsewhere (Palmer, 2001; 2013), one of the more powerful groups of actors in this policy network are 'cultural brokers'; that is, the occupational category who works the boundary between the production and consumption of cultural commodities such as sport and alcohol. Television and radio producers, journalists, public relations officers, marketing entrepreneurs and advertising agents, to name but a few, these brokers are part of an occupational group who specialise in the production and dissemination of symbolic goods and commodities – the very stuff of which both sport and alcohol are made. Working to produce (and profit from) the ideologies, images and resources of popular culture, these brokers have become an imperative class in contemporary times. As the anthropologist Ade Peace points out, brokers are both 'middlemen of renown and masters in the politics of cultural dissembling' (1998: 278).

In the cultural broker, we see the dovetailing of several different intellectual legacies. First, 'the broker' evokes Ewen's (1973) earlier conceptualisation of 'captains of consciousness', although Ewen reserves his term for brokers of the advertising industry. Second, the idea of the broker resonates with the notion of the 'cultural intermediary' coined by Bourdieu (1984), and third, the new cultural broker has come to assume the role of the 'power elite' first coined by C. Wright Mills (1956) more than 40 years ago. In a specifically sporting context, the notion of the broker is not incompatible with the idea of the 'sportsnet' popularised by Nixon (1993; 1996).

In terms of sport and alcohol policy-making, cultural brokers are intrinsically linked to the alcohol industry. In popular (and academic) parlance, 'the industry' has become something of a catch-all occupational category that encompasses a range of professions that deal with the production and consumption of alcohol. Including public relations officers, marketing entrepreneurs and advertising agents, the brokers of the sport-alcohol nexus play an increasingly central role in what the sport-alcohol nexus looks like. As Hawkins, Holden and McCambridge note in relation to UK alcohol policy, 'it has been widely claimed that the UK government has afforded too prominent a role to the alcohol industry in both the development and implementation of alcohol policy' (2012: 297).

What is imperative to note however, is that brokerage often requires processes of disguise, diversion and discursive manipulation. Much of the influence of the broker in production of the sport-alcohol nexus comes through in an entrepreneurial discourse which seeks to persuade the mass audience that the fruits of the brokers' labour will have particular public and personal benefits.

In terms of alcohol, these benefits can be three-fold. According to Mary Douglas (1987) alcohol performs three social tasks: first, it shows the world 'as it is'; second, drinking provides a model for social relationships by constructing an ideal world by defining relations between people. As argued elsewhere in the book, many of the perceived personal or social benefits are aspirational and, certainly, many of the messages of alcohol advertising emphasise fun, friendship or companionship, status (to return to some of the ideas of Bourdieu from Chapter 2) and connoisseurship (or how to enjoy fine wines and liquors). Importantly, most of these themes or the rationales that underpin them (notwithstanding connoisseurship) are indirect and suggest purchase by referencing something other than the alcohol itself.

It is in terms of Douglas' (1987) third function of drinking that the brokers of the sport-alcohol nexus become especially visible. For Douglas, the third function of drinking is an economic one, an observation echoed by Chzran. As Chrzan notes 'every society that uses alcohol creates economic structures for production, distribution and consumption, and alcohol usually provides significant revenue to producers and the state' (2012: 109). As we've seen elsewhere in the book, alcohol can bring considerable economic benefits to state and national or federal governments through measures such as the use of price and taxation and availability, perhaps ironically, those measured also recognised as being among the most effective evidence-based approaches to reducing alcohol-related harm.

It is this tension between the economic benefits of alcohol through sales and consumption and the need to restrict the economics of alcohol sales in order to minimise harm that enables the work of the cultural broker to come in to his or her own. Through alcohol advertising, in particular, we see that the practices of image manipulation and cultural management are central to the work of the cultural broker or intermediary. One of the creators of the Absolut Vodka brand, for example, states that:

> Basically, my profession is about invading peoples' integrity ... I get them interested in things they are not interested in, and I get them to long for things they didn't know existed. That is why it is fundamentally meaningless to ask people what they want (Hamilton, 1994: 102).

In other words, drug and alcohol policy, its governance, and its effects, is not simply the content of decisions and documents that are produced by politicians and bureaucrats. It also consists of the combination of individual interactions that take place within the framework provided by these instruments of power (Stevens, 2011: 402) and between the brokers so central to ensuring the circulation of power within the sport-alcohol nexus.

Consequences of policy-making

To return to the idea that policy is not a 'neutral' process but one that is always socially constructed; the product of considerable cultural work on the part of a whole range of individuals and organisations, including cultural brokers, this invites the question of what are the consequences (real or imagined) of the cultural work that underpins the construction of, in this case, alcohol policy?

As discussed already in the book, the discourse associated with harm minimisation in relation to alcohol consumption, is part of a 'proliferation of governmental directives for healthy living' (Keane, 2013: 151) in terms of eating and exercise, among other things, where there is a 'regulatory effect' on health discourses and practices whereby individuals are exhorted to make informed choices, to take responsibility for their wellbeing and to reduce their risks of future ill health (Peterson, Davis, Fraser and Lindsay, 2010). As Peterson, et al. state 'in the new public health, everyone is called upon to play their part in advancing the "public's health" through attention to lifestyle, healthy eating, exercise and preventative testing' (2010: 394).

In shifting the focus to 'the public' playing its part in the new public health, a key aim becomes to minimise (or at the very least, to appear to) the imposition of excessive top-down institutional approaches to policy-making, drawing instead on the symbolic work of cultural brokerage to use drinking to shows the world 'as it is' or a model for social relationships. In terms of healthy living and alcohol guidelines, the symbolic work undertaken by brokers invite active participation, personal investment and, often enough in the domain of health and wellbeing, some degree of self-sacrifice (Nettleton, 1997).

The three-fold functions of alcohol, when overlaid by a discussion of cultural brokerage enable a discussion of policy in all the contexts in which it is produced and practiced be that in the corridors of government, the pub or liquor store, the sports stadium or the after-match celebrations in the club rooms. While analyses of the sport-alcohol nexus and the issues of sponsorship and policy that sit within it tend to reify a harm minimisation approach, as I've suggested here, sociologists need to ask how this approach has come to be. What are the conditions of its existence, by which mechanisms is it produced and reproduced? By whom, and to what effect or consequence.

Conclusion

This chapter has explored the implications of two of the key practices which dominate much of the discourse and debates surrounding sports-associated drinking: issues of marketing and sponsorship and those of policy relating to health education, harm minimisation, licensing, taxation and regulation. These are often seen to sit in tension with one another in the sport-alcohol nexus. The central theme of this chapter, as it is for the book more broadly, is the importance of social context and cultural meanings in explaining drinking among particular sporting communities, and as I have argued in this chapter, context and meaning are key to developing and implementing policy across the spectrum from harm minimisation to industry regulation. As Esenbach-Stangl and Thom note, there is a need to recognise 'the importance of the cultural context and cultural sensitivity in developing policies and planning research' (2009: 14).

This focus on context and meaning reflects the broader shift in studies of alcohol and other drug use, particularly those interested in addiction, noted in Chapter 1. As I noted then, qualitative research has been useful for questioning the prevailing medical assumption throughout the 1950s and 1960s that drug addiction was a disease and drug users were 'passive, anxious and inadequate people' (Neale, et al., 2005: 1587), suggesting instead that drug addiction was a social experience that needed to be understood as an 'everyday' rather than deviant social practice. In this way, qualitative research has been instrumental in shaping policy and practice in relation to substance consumption.

Certainly, qualitative research was fundamental throughout the 1980s and 1990s in response to the global public health imperative to reduce HIV and other blood borne infections (Connell and Huggins, 1998; Connell, et al., 1991), along with users' experiences of service provision (Neale, 1988) and patient views of brief interventions in alcohol and primary health care (Lock, 2004). This research has all served as an instrumental starting point for seeking to understand the effectiveness (or not) of particular interventions and strategies aimed at harm minimisation in relation to excessive alcohol consumption, as it relates to sport or elsewhere.

There is no particular consensus regarding policy and practice responses, rather an emphasis on developing, as far as possible, evidence-based strategies and approaches which are culturally sensitive to national and local cultures and which take account of differences between different population groups.

More particularly, socio-cultural studies of alcohol use and misuse can bring a particular perspective to understandings of policy discourse, debate and action that comes some way to reconciling the tension between health promotion and the promotional culture of sponsorship, marketing and the governmental constraints of regulation. As I have suggested throughout the book, the sport-alcohol nexus is cut through with paradoxes and contradictions and the intersections between health promotion and the promotional culture of sport-related drinking brings this into particularly sharp relief.

Chapter 9
Rethinking Drinking and Sport

From the previous chapters, it should be evident that this book has been centrally concerned with the myriad, complex and contradictory ways in which the production and consumption of sport intersects with the production and consumption of alcohol. The book has essentially been about the 'sport-alcohol nexus'; that is the three-fold interplay between sport and alcohol in terms of: i) cultural practices and social identities; ii) pleasurable and problematic relationships to alcohol, and; iii) prevention, rehabilitation and culture change. That is, my interest has been in the ways in which sport-related drinking is understood, experienced and manifested as a set of social relationships, as a policy problem and as embedded in crucial narratives and practices of treatment and recovery. In adopting this focus, I have attempted to rethink drinking and sport; specifically, I have sought to extend the theoretical, conceptual and empirical base of studies of sport-related drinking so as to challenge many of the taken-for-granted orthodoxies from which research, policy and practice have often been developed.

The Rational Revisited

The starting point for the book was a concern with an overriding emphasis on male drinking that linked the consumption of alcohol to the cultural assertion of hegemonic masculinity. This, I suggested, had oriented the research agenda in very particular ways and, in doing so, had brought a pre-existing set of assumptions to the discussion that, when mobilised in media commentary, policy discussions and/or research agendas constructed the 'problem' of sport-related drinking in particular, pre-determined ways. While the social and policy problems associated with sport-related drinking are unquestionably very real and critical areas for on-going interrogation (and parts of the book have done this), my concern was not so much to engage with these debates or revisit the assumptions that underpin them, so much as to bring to our attention the kind of cultural practices and identities that have been obscured by foregrounding sport-related drinking as a bastion of masculinity. As I have explored here, women, non-drinkers, non-traditional drinkers, or drinkers in non-traditional sports have all been fruitful areas of sociological inquiry, as have 'athlete addicts' as well as those key workers and clients engaged with the delivery of sports-based interventions that seek to mitigate the costs and consequences of alcohol-related harms, particularly in terms of crime, violence and social disorder.

In much the same way, I was keen to explore alternative theoretical frameworks through which sport-related drinking might be explained, interpreted or analysed so as to complement (or contradict) the default theoretical perspectives that view sport-related drinking through a gender lens, and that position sports-associated drinking as an exemplar of hegemonic masculinity or, where it involves women, that frames their behaviours as challenging or subverting normative notions of femininity. Indeed, a central aim of the book has been to reconsider, expand and extend some of the concepts and ideas that have emerged from previous theorising about drug-taking. As I explored in Chapters 2 and 3, concepts such as determined drunkenness, governmentality, symbolic capital and hegemonic drinking can all help ground an analysis of sport-related drinking in terms of cultural practices, social meanings and lived experiences in ways that complement analyses of sport and drinking as normative, gendered social practices. This, by no means, is to deny that sport, and drinking, can be highly gendered activities. However, as I have suggested throughout the book, there is considerably more to the sport-alcohol nexus than the production and reproduction of normative gendered behaviours, and the primary focus of the book has been to challenge some of the existing orthodoxies and taken-for-granted positions that surround sports-associated drinking.

Given that there is no shortage of analyses of sport or alcohol in relation to gender and masculinity, it was not my intention add to this substantial literature, mindful of Houlihan's warning that 'there is always a temptation among social scientists to overextend and analyse a concept until it dies of exhaustion' (1994: 372). My intention instead was to attempt to broaden thinking about sport-related drinking, drawing particularly on other ways of engaging with the debates about alcohol consumption that underpin scholarly thinking on drinking more widely. I was particularly concerned with both the 'everyday' and the 'exceptional' nature of sport-related drinking; that is, how alcohol intersects with and inflects sport as a promotional activity, as a cultural practice, as a social and policy problem and as a site of meaning, representation and identity.

In foregrounding the everyday, sometimes mundane, sometimes extreme and exceptional ways in which sport-related drinking is understood, experienced and manifested as a set of social relationships, as a policy problem and as embedded in narratives and practices of treatment and recovery, at one and the same time, the book took a particular shape or tenor. My interest was, fundamentally, to challenge the taken-for-granted assumptions that surround sport-related drinking in order to address some of the theoretical and methodological gaps in academic approaches to studies of sport and alcohol. My central argument has been that this challenge is long overdue, for sociologists of sport, in particular, are 'at risk of simply reproducing stereotypes and assumptions of sport-related drinking more common to popular accounts, instead of developing critical, theoretically informed analyses of drinking and sport that are must be our key point of difference' (Palmer, 2013a: 2).

In being principally concerned with the everyday (as well as the exceptional) contexts of alcohol use, I have advocated throughout for the need for more nuanced and critical socio-cultural perspectives on alcohol consumption in relation to sport that can inform and influence theory, policy and practice. Moreover, my interest in sport-related drinking as an everyday social practice that is shared predominantly by ordinary people in mainstream population groups sought to shift the focus away from some of the more vulnerable communities who are frequently marginalised and stigmatised for their drug and alcohol use. While not intending that the book be read as anything close to resembling a comparison between everyday or 'normal' drinkers and drinking behaviours and those that sit at the margins, the point remains that drunkenness and the manifold social, economic and medical problems that it involves, may be understood better if seen in relation to a culture or a community's 'normal' way of drinking.

To this end, Chapter 2, in particular, put forward some alternative theoretical perspectives for understanding and explaining sport-related drinking that represent the 'ongoing need to reassess and reinvigorate the theoretical frameworks that drive drug research, policy and practice' (Moore, 2006: 324). Notions of 'calculated hedonism' (Szmigin, et al., 2008) and 'serious leisure' (Stebbins, 1992; 2001) used elsewhere in the social sciences to discuss drinking and leisure and consumption practices, offered two particular conceptual frameworks that have been overlooked when theorising the social practices that surround *sport*-related drinking cultures and behaviours. Similarly, theories of governmentality and normalisation that have been used elsewhere in studies of alcohol and other drugs have not been applied to analyses of sport-related drinking, and the book outlined some possible research avenues that could be explored to this effect. As I have asserted elsewhere 'a more nuanced engagement with a wider range of theoretical frameworks might help better understand and explain the diversity and complexity of drinkers and drinking in sport' (Palmer, 2013a: 2).

Turning then to the more empirical chapters, Chapters 3 and 4 drew on a series of perhaps counter-intuitive case studies to illustrate some of the myriad articulations in the sport-alcohol nexus. Focussing on both female drinkers and the attitudes of women to sport-related drinking in the context of Australian football, non-drinkers in sport, non-traditional drinkers and drinking in non-traditional sports, such as Ultimate Frisbee, snowboarding and roller derby, allowed an exploration of the intersectoral connections between age, class, gender, ethnicity, place and location, as well as gender, and how this plays out in the sport-alcohol nexus. In other words, this way of framing sport-related drinking in terms of 'gender plus' can help sharpen our analytical focus and open up new areas of inquiry (and urgency) for research, policy and practice.

Building on this, Chapter 6 examined some of the strategies and initiatives that sporting clubs and community-based organisation have in place to address, recognise and change the 'culture of drinking' in sport, while Chapter 7 explored the paradoxical and contradictory ways in which sports-based interventions have been used to prevent or mitigate against the harms related to alcohol misuse. Here, I sought to examine the ways in which sport is offered up as a key intervention in recovery, rehabilitation and desistance from many of the health and social costs and consequences associated with alcohol misuse. Following Coalter (2007; 2013a; 2013b) and others, I have been critical of the 'mythopoeic' nature of sport and the ways in which it is widely promoted as a panacea for a range of social ills, in this case, harms related to alcohol misuse. My voice has joined that of others calling for a more rigorous use of evidence (both qualitative and quantitative) to demonstrate (or not) the extent to which the kinds of sports-based interventions described in Chapters 6 and 7 actually improve outcomes for their clients. As Haudenyhuyse, Theebom and Nols note, there is a need to evaluate outcomes in terms of biographical, institutional and political competencies for it is 'argued that there is an acute need for re-socialising sports research regarding social interventions for socially vulnerable groups' (2012: 471).

A broader empirical and theoretical understanding of sport and alcohol also raises questions for an emergent policy agenda, particularly, but not exclusively in terms of health and social issues. As I argued throughout the book, there is a need for wider engagement with social science concepts to generate a theoretically informed framework for understanding the processes of policy-making, and its constructed and contested nature. Indeed, a key theme developed is that policy is the product of considerable cultural work on the part of a whole range of individuals and organisations, and this has significant implications for the management, administration and governance of alcohol policy as it relates particularly to sport.

As I have argued throughout, an expanded sociological research agenda on sport-related drinking can help inform policy-related issues and debates in ways that are increasingly being recognised by policy makers (and sociologists) in alcohol and other drugs fields more broadly. This is particularly the case when attempting to implement policy related to alcohol misuse among young people: as Eisnebach-Stangl and Thom note 'to understand youthful binge drinking and associated behaviours, and to find ways of intervening to prevent or reduce harm, it is necessary to understand the prevailing concept(s) of acceptable and unacceptable forms of intoxication and intoxicated behaviours and its/their wider social and cultural determinants' (2009: 1).

My fairly fluid engagement with a range of issues and debates also meant I adopted a fairly fluid approach to my interpretation of the sport-alcohol nexus. Throughout, I have used the terms 'sport-related drinking' and 'sports-associated drinking' fairly interchangeably. I chose these terms deliberately so as to capture the diversity and, to some extent, the ambiguity of the behaviours and practices that the book has principally been concerned with. Equally, the 'interstitial' (Bhabba, 2004: 3) nature of sport-related drinking – encompassing many sports and intersecting with a range of social problems and policy contexts (crime, health, governance, licensing and legislation, and so on) – meant my approach to writing the book focussed on no single sport, sporting code or cultural or geographical context.

That said, while the focus, in the main, was on the drinking practices and their consequences as experienced, understood and enacted by sportsmen/women and by sports fans, the book was also, although less so, concerned with those affected by another's sport-related drinking, and the second half of the book, in particular, explored some of the damage(s) done by another's sport-related drinking in a broader context of stigma, shame, violence, abuse, treatment and recovery. This relatively fluid understanding of the nature and extent of sport-related drinking also highlighted its problematic and paradoxical features, particularly in the context of industry promotion, regulation, governance and legislation, which provide the broader social and policy backdrop to much of the book.

Although 'anyone involved in sport, whether as a player or as a fan, will almost inevitably be exposed to a strong message that alcohol and sport are inextricably linked' (Jones, Phillipson and Lynch, 2006: n.p), I could not, and did not, hope to cover all aspects of sport-related drinking. My focus has been primarily on the *social contexts* of sport-related drinking. As I have argued throughout, the sociality of sport-related drinking, like drinking elsewhere, is dependent on culture and context. Sports-associated drinking, like other forms of drinking, does not take place 'just anywhere', and I have adopted the position that sport-related drinking is essentially a social act that is subject to a variety of rules and norms regarding who may drink what, when, where, why, how, with whom, and so on. This has inevitably skewed the focus away from biological, biocultural and biophysical accounts of alcohol consumption. Certainly, this work on patterns and prevalence, and the physiological or psychological effects of alcohol consumption can add value to socio-cultural studies, but, because I do not work in this field, I have referred to this research somewhat tangentially. The social rather than the individual, and the contextual rather than the pathological, has been the lens through which I've framed much of the analysis presented.

Indeed, the book has been rooted in a focus on the 'definitions of the situation' (Thomas, 1937 in Herman-Kinney and Kinney, 2012: 4) in which sport-related drinking occurs. Borrowing from Jayne, et al., my argument throughout has been that if studies of sport-related drinking are to fully capture the meaning and importance of drinking, then 'the interpenetration of practices and processes related to production, consumption, regulation, representation and identity must be fully investigated' (2006: 452). Thus, the book has been grounded in empirical, largely qualitative research that could give voice and meaning to the everyday contexts of sport-related drinking, its pleasures, its harms, its impacts and its consequences.

In particular, I was concerned to include competing and under-represented views within broader debates about the cultures and consequences of sport-related drinking. For this reason, Chapters 3 and 4 were empirical studies of drinking among female drinkers associated with Australian sport, non-drinkers in an environment where strong normative codes of hegemonic drinking prevail and, drinkers in non-traditional sporting contexts. While there is a rich literature on the socially constructed and constitutive nature of drinking, this has tended to focus on particular sports (predominantly football across all codes). My interest in Chapters 3 and 4 was as much with what people *don't do* as much as with developing different frameworks for making sense of what we know already. That is, I was keen to ask questions of what we don't know.

Framing up counter-intuitive examples that may help sharpen our analyses and focus our conceptual lenses is at the heart of much of my intellectual project in this book and, indeed, my research interests more widely. That said, there is considerably more to be done here. Chapters 3 and 4 started to raise some questions in relation to forms of masculinity that sit outside of the trope of orthodox or hegemonic masculinity – older men, gay men, men from outside of the major metropoles in the Global North – but what of older women, lesbians or women from outside of the major metropoles in the Global North? The glossing of the broad categories of gender, age and sexuality notwithstanding, such counter-intuitive examples of drinking and sport provide a useful starting point for further nuanced, fine-grained empirical research.

Relatedly, while the use of illegal drugs in sport – for either recreation or to enhance performance – has been the subject of considerable scholarly debate and media and public scrutiny, this has not been my concern here. I have written elsewhere about drugs in sport (Palmer, 2000; 2014), and certainly there are some similarities in the discourse of ethics and entitlement that accompany drug-taking and dangerous levels of alcohol consumption by athletes. That said, the use of recreational drugs and/or prescription medicines by some athletes is worth noting as, anecdotally at least, it appears that some are turning to these forms of 'highs' to escape club-enforced penalties if caught consuming alcohol during the playing season. In other words, it is far easier to get caught with a drink in your hand than if you've swallowed a small pill in the privacy of your own home, and athletes are seeking to evade scrutiny and the risk of a 'fall from grace' if caught.

The Ethics of Research with Alcohol

One of the things I have not explicitly addressed in the book, yet it remains something of the elephant in the room, is the question of research ethics when conducting social research with individuals and communities where alcohol is consumed. Drinking alcohol can, as Donnelly (2013) notes, have significant consequences for both research participants and researchers in the field, so some concluding reflections and observations are worth making here.

Given the subject and nature of my research – qualitative, ethnographic inquiry with people who drink, often heavily, and who frequently drink to get drunk – I am often required by university ethics boards and, more fundamentally, by my own commitment to sound research practice to think through the pragmatic realities, risks and potential consequences of the work I do for myself, and for the individuals and communities whose lives and experiences inform my research. As I have written about elsewhere (Palmer and Thompson, 2010), the sport-alcohol nexus can be a vexed research field. Issues such as consent, confidentiality, disclosure, privacy or betrayal, along with female researchers entering into predominantly male sporting environments in which alcohol is routinely (and often excessively) consumed all pose a particular set of dilemmas, as do the potential dangers of conducting research with participants who are inebriated and the duty-of-care to research participants. While I do not wish to revisit these arguments at length here, 'a failure to attend to these and other risks and dilemmas can threaten the viability of research among drinking-based communities and subcultures' (Palmer and Thompson, 2010: 421).

The key ethical concerns for me, as a researcher, and, it seems, for university ethics boards, are the question of whether to consume alcohol, the notion of informed consent where research subjects are impaired, and the issue of duty-of-care. While individual researchers may negotiate these questions differently, and reach their own conclusions as to their position on what kind of behaviours or approaches to research are appropriate to their own circumstances, working and writing in fields where alcohol (or other drugs) is consumed does demand a level of critical reflection on entering, being in, and exiting the fieldwork setting.

As a social researcher, it has been imperative to be entirely transparent about my purpose for visiting sporting matches and spending time in the various contexts and settings where drinking takes place. Like other research where gaining and maintaining access depends on good relations with gatekeepers and respondents (Sampson and Thomas, 2003; Belousov, et al., 2007), my research is openly presented as being 'for a book about sport and drinking' and to support such professional claims, I always carried university identification.

Drinking alcohol can carry with it certain perceptions of moral judgment, and a researcher being seen to drink alcohol often provides a crucial point of entry into the culture of alcohol that he or she may be interested in learning more about. For me, 'drinking on the job' exposed me to many of the practices associated with drinking, and the consumption of alcohol became fundamental to the research process in terms of the access it granted me and the ways in which it then legitimated my presence in the field.

My visible alcohol consumption was a deliberate research strategy to facilitate my fieldwork. It offset the perception that I was taking the moral high ground and it provided direct and intimate access to the very attitudes, behaviours and practices I had been commissioned to document and detail. In this respect, it would have been less appropriate to abstain than to indulge. Nonetheless, I needed to approach my alcohol consumption with some degree of care to ensure I could carry out my fieldwork unimpaired, and I have detailed this at length elsewhere (Palmer and Thompson, 2010). My involvement with participants who regularly drank to excess opened up a number of professional dilemmas and ethical concerns to do with informed consent and my duty-of-care in relation to those participants who were under the influence of alcohol. As other researchers have also experienced (Gee, 2013; Donnelly, 2013), it is sometimes necessary to take part in activities and events with people who are clearly intoxicated. This gives rise to some particular ethical issues regarding informed consent.

It is one of the fundamental tenets of social research that participants in research projects are fully informed of the purpose, potential harms, likely benefits and, indeed, what their involvement in the research will entail. There is thus a responsibility on the researcher to explain and to make sure participants have fully understood the purpose, procedures and potential harms and benefits of the research. Issues of communication and comprehension become more complicated when conducting research with groups or individuals whose ability to make an informed decision about participation is compromised, and there is a body of literature that explores these issues in relation to young children, people with disability or people with mental health issues.

In terms of my own research, I have encountered people who are so intoxicated that their ability to give informed consent is profoundly compromised. In those cases where I have been unsure of a subject's ability to understand what we were doing or to appreciate the implications of my notebook, tape recorder or camera, I took the decision not to record data. As Dewalt, et al. note:

> It is the ethnographer's responsibility not only to think a bit first, but to make conscious decisions on what to report and what to decline to report based on careful consideration of the ethical dimensions of the impact of the information on those who provide it, and the goals of the research (1998: 273).

While I observed and noted the context and ways in which obviously drunk people were drinking, I did not seek personal or individual information in those instances where I was doubtful that informed consent could be given. While it could be argued that because much of what was being observed was already in the public domain, then obtaining informed consent was not necessary, I felt it both invasive and exploitative to observe, photograph and then record for a wider audience people who were quite clearly incapacitated through alcohol. Thus, attempts to obtain consent to be interviewed, photographed or observed were made wherever possible.

The ability to give informed consent was determined by the tell-tale indicators of slurred speech, an unsteady gait, bloodshot eyes or, more simply, the confession that a person was 'shit-faced'. While open to considerable interpretation, such judgements still gave me a degree of confidence that participants had not taken part in something they might regret. The rise of the ubiquitous 'selfie'; that is a photograph taken of oneself and posted onto social media sites in the public domain raises further questions as to the legitimacy of these images as research texts and sources.

Being in environments where heavy drinking is commonplace has also given me pause for thought as to issues of a duty-of-care to those who are drinking. My research teams have deliberated at length about what, if any, our responsibilities are to people who are clearly intoxicated in terms of their own (and others) safety. After much consideration, our general position has been that our responsibilities to intoxicated people are no more or less than they are in a non-research setting (such as having a drink with a friend in a bar where someone was clearly drunk), and it is not in our remit to intervene. Our rationale for this is that the intoxication is not a result of participation in the research, but is an integral part of the culture that often orients the research in the first instance. Following Sugden's guiding principle that researchers are not agent provocateurs, 'we should not set in motion procedures which otherwise would not have happened in order to unearth interesting material' (1997: 243); we did not initiate action or intervene in events as they unfolded. Even so, the unpredictability of social research is made more so with the unpredictability that alcohol consumption can bring and calls for a particular kind of researcher reflexivity and 'sense-checking' before, during and after the research engagement.

Contradictions and Paradoxes

Along with my concern with the overriding emphasis on male drinking that linked the consumption of alcohol to the cultural assertion of hegemonic masculinity, part of my reason for writing this book was what I saw to be the inherently paradoxical and contradictory nature of the relationship between sport and alcohol. On the one hand, the 'problem' of sport-related drinking is well documented, particularly in popular accounts of high profile sportsmen being implicated in accounts of sexual abuse and other forms of violence, and I have traced out some of the media and popular discourse around this, as well as some of the culture change strategies and initiatives adopted by clubs and organisations to tackle the problem of sport-related drinking, and the need for image or brand management that often accompanies a very public 'fall from grace'.

At the same time, sport, in narratives elsewhere, is presented, not as a problem, but as a panacea. That is, it provides an opportunity for recovery and rehabilitation from many of the social problems associated with alcohol-related harms, where sport is used in prevention and treatment programme for clients, usually young people, who are at risk of drug and alcohol misuse. This tension or contradiction is not easily reconciled, yet pursuing some of the questions it invites or obscures is an important step towards challenging popular assumptions about sport-related drinking that cast and limit understandings of alcohol in sport in very particular ways.

Certainly, sport-related drinking is implicated in a whole host of health and social problems and is enjoyed by particular kinds of men, in particular kinds of settings that do little to counter the dominant stereotype I began this book with. However, the fundamental point here is that there are *other* relationships that men and women have to sport, and to alcohol, as athletes and as consumers of sport (and alcohol), and these are yet to be fully realised in sociological analyses of sports-related drinking, whilst being attended to in other social science accounts of drinking beyond sport. The pleasure of drinking and its implications for policy, health, governance and regulation, female drinkers, non-drinkers in sporting codes where strong normative codes of drinking exist, and the relationships between locational disadvantage, alcohol consumption and sport, are just some of the areas that are yet to be fully explored in sociological treatments of sport-related drinking. Looking to alternative explanatory frameworks beyond those we routinely employ can help widen the empirical and theoretical bases through which we can understand and explain drinking and drinkers in sport.

Highlighting these new areas of sociological inquiry does raise a potential concern over competing and contemporaneous paradigms, and whether we are talking about aspects of social behaviour that cannot be reconciled by theorising them differently. This, for me, is a 'yes, but … ' problem. That is, yes, the behaviours and practices associated with sport-related drinking can continue to be explained through theories oriented by concerns with gender, for example, but there are other ways in which this can be done as well. Recognising that fun and pleasure are legitimate sources of meaning does not detract from broader issues for health, social policy, governance and regulation. Indeed, the hedonism of particular kinds of drinking, be that in relation to sport or anything else, presents club officials, governing bodies and policy makers with a dilemma, for it clashes with other expectations of citizens, including notions of responsibility, reasonableness and self-control, and negotiating the tensions and contradictions inherent in the pleasure of drinking raises a whole set of questions for research, policy and practice.

Drawing attention to new relationships to alcohol and sport, and suggesting alternative ways of analysing and interpreting them, is not to dismiss established conceptual paradigms. New theories and explanatory frameworks do not detract from the value of past approaches, but their relative absence does suggest a need to widen our frame of vision so as to develop a more fully realised sociological understanding of sport-related drinking. Moreover, developing a fuller understanding of the diversity and complexity of drinking in the context of sport, through the kind of research agenda outlined here, can usefully inform policy debates and developments around alcohol use and misuse.

Finally

The previous chapters have, in essence, sketched out a mandate of sorts for rethinking drinking and sport. While sport has provided the empirical basis for the book, the themes and debates it has engaged with are of relevance to studies of drinking (or other drugs) in other empirical contexts and settings. In attempting to broaden out our understandings of the myriad, complex and contradictory ways in which the production and consumption of sport intersects with the production and consumption of alcohol, I have attempted to both ask and respond to a series of questions through which to interrogate the sport-alcohol nexus through a somewhat revitalised theoretical, empirical and conceptual framework.

These guiding questions or principles may include:

- an on-going commitment to identify new (and recurrent) research problems in studies of sport-related drinking;

- the importance of reflecting on, critiquing and debating the ethical and methodological aspects of empirical research where alcohol is consumed;
- an openness to identify new empirical bases and theoretical perspectives through which to engage in broader debates over the role of alcohol in constructing sporting identities beyond those that are gender based);
- contributing to debates that focus on the role of alcohol in reproducing health promoting and health damaging behaviours, as well as;
- adding to the evidence base that can better inform research, policy and practice.

As a site for social research, sport-related drinking is empirically rich and conceptually diverse, and studies of alcohol consumption are nothing short of ethnographic gold. Alcohol use makes visible all kinds of social relationships, articulations and tensions between individual bodies and global markets, or between inner and out worlds. As Chzran puts it: 'drinking is a deeply cultural act' (2013: 5). Understanding the social contexts and uses of alcohol, in relation to sport or elsewhere, helps us to understand the demands upon people's lives, the complexities of leisure and work, to juggle competing demands, and to manage stress, pain, illness or despair. Studies of the everyday and exceptional ways in which alcohol is consumed allow us to explore the boundaries and connections between physical and emotional worlds, the desire for physical pleasure, the problems this presents for policy and practice, and the tensions of indulgence and abstinence and between risk and regulation. The questions that can be both posed and answered by rethinking drinking, in this case, as it relates to sport, provide a unique point of entry into our collective social and historical biography.

Bibliography

ABC (2013) Dwarf entertainer allegedly set on fire in St Kilda 'Mad Monday' event. Available at: <www.abc.net.au/news/2013-09-03/dwarf-entertainer-allegedly-set-on-fire-in-st-kilda-27mad-mond/4930858> (accessed 8 January 2014).

Abdul Razak, M., Omar-Fauzee., M. and Abd-Latif R. (2010) The perspective of Arabic Muslim women toward sport participation. *Journal of Asia Pacific Studies* 1(2): 364–77.

Adams, T. (1998) *Addicted*. London: Collins Willlow.

Adams, A., Anderson, E. and McCormack, M. (2010) Establishing and challenging masculinity: The influence of gendered discourses in organized sport. *Journal or Language and Social Psychology* 29(3): 278–300.

Agar, M. (2003) Towards a qualitative epidemiology. *Qualitative Health Research* 13(7): 974–86.

Agar, M. (1973) *Ripping and running: A formal ethnography of urban heroin addicts*. New York: Seminar Press.

Ahmad, A. (2011) British football: Where are the Muslim female footballers? *Soccer and Society* 12(3): 443–56.

Alaszewski, A. (2011) Drugs, risk and society: Government, governance or governmentality? *Health, Risk & Society* 13(5): 389–96.

Aldridge, J., Measham, F. and Williams, L. (2011) *Illegal leisure revisited: Changing patterns of alcohol and drug use in adolescents and young adults*. London: Routledge.

Allen-Collinson, J. and Hockey, J. (2005) Autoethnography: Self Indulgence or Rigorous Methodology. In M. McNamee (ed.) *Philosophy and the sciences of exercise, health and sport: Critical perspectives on research methods*. London: Routledge, pp. 187–202.

Allen-Collinson, J. and Hockey, J. (2007) 'Working out' Identity: Distance runners and the management of disrupted identity. *Leisure Studies* 26(4): 381–98.

Altheide, D.L. (1996) *Qualitative media analysis*. Thousand Oaks, CA: Sage.

Anderson, E. (2009) *Inclusive masculinity: The changing nature of masculinities*. New York: Routledge.

Anderson, E. (2005) *In the game: Gay athletes and the cult of masculinity*. Albany: State University of New York Press.

Anderson, E., McCormack., M. and Lee, H. (2012) Male team sport hazing initiations in a culture of decreasing homohysteria. *Journal of Adolescent Research* 27(4): 427–48.

Anderson, L. and Taylor, J. (2010) Standing out while fitting in: Serious leisure identities and aligning actions among skydivers and gun collectors. *Journal of Contemporary Ethnography* 39(1): 34–59.

Archetti, E. (2001) The spectacle of a heroic life: Diego Maradona. In D. Andrews and S. Jackson (eds) *Sport stars: The cultural politics of sporting celebrities.* London: Routledge, pp. 151–63.

Armstrong, G. and Hognestad, H. (2006) Hitting the bar: Alcohol, football identities and global flows in Norway. In T. Wilson (ed.) *Food, drink and identity in Europe.* Amsterdam: Rodopi, pp. 85–110.

Armstrong. G. (1993) ' … Like that Desmond Morris?' In D. Hobbs and T. May (eds) *Interpreting the field.* Oxford: Oxford University Press, pp. 3–44.

Armstrong, L. (2000) *It's not about the bike: My journey back to life.* New York: Putman.

Atkinson, A.M., Kirton, A. and Sumall, H.R. (2012) The gendering of alcohol in consumer magazines: An analysis of male and female targeted publications. *Journal of Gender Studies* 21(4): 365–86.

Atkinson, M. (2009) Parkour, anarcho-environmentalism, and poiesis. *Journal of Sport and Social Issues* 33(2): 169–94.

Atkinson, M. (2008) Triathlon, suffering and exciting significance. *Leisure Studies* 27(2): 165–80.

Australian Drug Foundation (ADF) (2002) *Good sports accreditation program.* Melbourne: Australian Drug Foundation.

Australian Institute of Health and Welfare (2011). *Statistics on drug use in Australia 2010.* Canberra: Australian Institute of Health and Welfare. Available at: <http://www.aihw.gov.au/publications/phe/sdua02/sdua02.pdf> (accessed 7 March 2011).

Ayers, T.C. and Treadwell, J. (2012) Bars, drugs and football thugs: Alcohol, cocaine use and violence in the night time economy among English football firms. *Criminology & Criminal Justice* 12(1): 93–100.

Babor, T., Caetano, R., Casswell, S., Edwards, G., Geisbrecht, N., Graham, K. et al. (2010) *Alcohol: No ordinary commodity.* 2nd edition. Oxford: Oxford University Press.

Babor, T., Caetano, R., Casswell, S., Edwards, G., Geisbrecht, N., Graham, K., et al. (2003) *Alcohol: No ordinary commodity.* In *Research and public policy.* New York: Oxford University Press.

Baum, F. (2008) *The new public health.* Abigdon: Oxford University Press.

BBC News (2012a) Beer 'Must be Sold' at Brazil World Cup, says Fifa. Available at: <http://www.bbc.co.uk/news/world-latin-america-16624823> (accessed 19 January 2012).

BBC News (2012b) Brazil World Cup beer law signed by President Rousseff, 6 June 2012. Available at: <http://www.bbc.com/news/world-latin-america-18348012?print=true> (accessed 7 April 2014).

Beasley, C. (2008) Rethinking masculinity in a globalizing world. *Men and Masculinities* 11(1): 86–103.

Beccaria, F. and Sande, A. (2003) Drinking games and rite of life projects: A social comparison of the meaning and functions of your people's use of alcohol during the rite of passage to adulthood in Italy and Norway. *Young. Nordic Journal of Youth Studies* 11(2): 99–119.

Beck, U. (1992) *Risk society: Towards a new modernity.* London: Sage.

Belousov, K., Horlick-Jones, T., Bloor, M., et al. (2007) Any port in a storm: Fieldwork difficulties in dangerous and crisis-ridden settings. *Qualitative Research* 7(2): 155–75.

Berridge, K. and Robinson T. (2011) Drug addiction as incentive sensitization. In. J. Poland and G. Graham (eds) *Addiction and responsibility.* Cambridge, MA: The MIT Press, pp. 21–53.

Berwick, B., Mulhern., B., Barkham, M., et al. (2008) Changes in undergraduate student alcohol consumption as they progress through university. *BMC Public Health* 8(163): 1–8.

Best, D. and Laudet, A. (2010) *The potential of recovery capital.* London: Royal Society for the Arts.

Bhaba, H. (2004) Statement for the critical inquiry symposium. *Critical Inquiry* 30(2): 342–9.

Biernacki, P. (1986) *Pathways from heroin addiction recovery without treatment.* Philadelphia, PA: Temple University Press.

Black, D., Lawson, J. and Fleishman, S. (1999) Excessive alcohol use by non-elite sportsmen. *Drug and Alcohol Review* 18(2): 201–5.

Blackman, S. (2007) 'Hidden ethnography': Crossing emotional borders in qualitative accounts of young people's lives. *Sociology* 41(4): 699–716.

Blackshaw, T. and Crabbe, T. (2004) *New perspectives on sport and 'deviance': Consumption, performativity and social control.* Cambridge: Polity Press.

Blake, M. (2012) No more booze for Bombers, *The Age*, Tuesday 27 March. Available at: <http://www.theage.com.au/afl/afl-news/no-more-booze-for-bombers-20120326-1vuo6.html> (accessed 10 May 2015).

Bloomfield K., Gmel, G., Neve, R. and Mustonen, H. (2001) Investigating gender convergence in alcohol consumption in Finland, Germany, the Netherlands and Switzerland. *Substance Abuse* 22: 39–54.

Bourdieu, P. (1989) Social space and symbolic power. *Sociological Theory* 7: 14–25.

Bourdieu, P. (1984) *Distinction: A social critique of the judgment of taste.* New York: Routledge and Kegan Paul.

Bourgois, P. (2002) Anthropology and epidemiology on drugs: The challenges of cross-methodological and theoretical dialogue. *International Journal of Drug Policy* 13(4): 259–69.

Bourgois, P. (2000) Disciplining addictions: The biopolitics of methadone and heroin in the United States. *Culture, Medicine & Psychiatry* 24(2): 165–95.

Bourgois, P. (1999) Theory, method and power in drug and HIV prevention research: A participant-observer's critique. *Substance Use and Misuse* 34(14): 2155–72.

Borgen, A. (2011) Gender and alcohol: The Swedish press debate. *Journal of Gender Studies* 20(2): 155–69.

Brady, M. (1992) Ethnography and understanding of Aboriginal drinking. *Journal of Drug Issues* 22(3): 699–712.

Brain, K. (2000) *Youth, alcohol and the emergence of the postmodern order.* Occasional Paper. Institute of Alcohol Studies: London.

Brown, R. and Gregg, M. (2012) The pedagogy of regret: Facebook, binge drinking and young women. *Continuum. Journal of Media & Cultural Studies* 26(3): 357–69.

Burdsey, D. (2011) *Race, ethnicity and football: Persisting debates and emergent Issues.* Routledge Research in Sport, Culture and Society. London: Routledge.

Burdsey, D. (2010) British Muslim experiences in English first-class cricket. *International Review for the Sociology of Sport* 45(3): 315–34.

Burdsey, D. (2004) 'One of the lads'? Dual ethnicity and assimilated ethnicities in the careers of British Asian professional footballers. *Ethnic and Racial Studies* 27 (5): 757–79.

Burdsey, D. and Randhawa, K. (2012) How can professional football clubs create welcoming and inclusive stadia for British Asian fans? *Journal of Policy Research in Tourism, Leisure and Events* 4(1): 105–11.

Butler, J. (2004) *Undoing gender.* London: Routledge.

Campbell, H. (2000) The glass phallus: Pub(lic) masculinity and drinking in rural New Zealand. *Rural Sociology* 65(4): 562–81.

Campbell, R. (2010) Staging globalization for national projects: Global sport markets and elite athletic transnational labor in Qatar. *International Review for the Sociology of Sport* 46(1): 45–60.

Cameron, D., Thomas, M., Madden, S., et al. (2000) Intoxicated across Europe: In search of meaning. *Addiction Research* 8(3): 233–42.

Caparo, R. (2000) Why college men drink: Alcohol, adventure and the paradox of masculinity. *Journal of American College Health* 48: 307–15.

Carless, D. and Douglas, K. (2008) Narrative, identity and mental health: How men with serious mental illness re-story their lives through sport and exercise. *Psychology of Sport and Exercise* 9(5): 576–94.

Carpenter, R., Fishlock., A., Mulroy., A., et al. (2008) After 'Unit 1421': An exploratory study into female students' attitudes and behaviours towards binge drinking at Leeds University. *Journal of Public Health* 30(1): 8–1.

Casey, M., Harvey, J., Eime, R. and Payne, W. (2012) Examining changes in the organisational capacity and sport-related health promotion policies. *Annals of Leisure Research* 15(3): 261–76.

Casswell, S. and Maxwell, A. (2005) What works to reduce alcohol-related harm and why aren't the policies more popular? *Social Policy Journal of New Zealand* 25: 118–41.

Chzran, J. (2013) *Alcohol: Social drinking in cultural context.* London: Routledge.

Clarkson, J.P., Giles-Corti, B., Donovan, R.J. and Frizzell, S.K. (2002) Play Hard Drink Safe: A pilot project to promote responsible alcohol consumption in sporting clubs in Western Australia. *Health Promotion Journal of Australia* 13(3): 226–31.

Clayton, B. (2012) Initiate: Constructing the 'reality' of male team sport initiation rituals. *International Review for the Sociology of Sport* 48(2): 204–19.

Clayton, B. and Harris, J. (2008) Our friend Jack: Alcohol, friendship and masculinity in university football. *Annals of Leisure Research* 11(3–4): 311–30.

Coakley, J. (2011) Youth sports: What counts as 'positive development?' *Journal of Sport and Social Issues* 35(3): 306–24.

Coalter, F. (2013a) *Sport for development: What game are we playing?* London: Routledge.

Coalter, F. (2013b) 'There is loads of relationships here': Developing a programme theory for sport-for-change programs. *International Review for the Sociology of Sport* 48(5): 594–612.

Coalter, F. (2007) *A wider social role for sport: Who's keeping score?* Abigdon, VA: Routledge.

Coalter, F., Allison, M. and Taylor, J. (2000) *The role of sport in regenerating deprived urban areas*. Edinburgh: Scottish Executive.

Coffey, A. (1999) *The ethnographic self: Fieldwork and the representation of identity*. London: Sage.

Collins, T. and Vamplew, W. (2002) *Mud, sweat and beers: A cultural history of Sport and Alcohol*. Oxford: Berg Publishers.

Collins, M., Henry, I., Houlihan, B., et al. (1999) *Sport and Social Inclusion: A Report to the Department of Culture, Media and Sport.*

Connell, R.W. (1995) *Masculinities*. Berkeley: University of California Press.

Connell, R. (1987) *Gender and power: Society, the person and sexual politics*. Cambridge: Polity Press.

Connell, R.W. and Messerchmidt, J.W. (2005) Hegemonic masculinity: Rethinking the concept. *Gender & Society* 19(6): 829–59.

Connell, R.W. and Huggins, A. (1998) Men's health. *Medical Journal of Australia* 169: 295–29.

Connell, R.W., Dowsett, G.W., Rodden, P. Davis, M., Watson, L. and Baxter, D. (1991) Social class, gay men, and AIDS prevention. *Australian Journal of Public Health* 15(3): 178–89.

Connor, J., Kydd, R., Shield, K. and Rehm, J. (2013) *Alcohol-attributable burden of disease and injury in New Zealand: 2004 and 2007.* Research report commissioned by the Health Promotion Agency. Wellington: Health Promotion Agency.

Connor, J., Broad, J., Rehm, J., Vander Hoorn, S. and Jackson, R. (2005) The burden of death, disease, and disability due to alcohol in New Zealand. *New Zealand Medical Journal* 118(1213).

Coveney, J. (2004) A qualitative study exploring socio-economic differences in parental lay knowledge of food and health: implications for public health nutrition. *Public Health Nutrition* 8:290–97.

Coveney, J. and Bunton, R. (2003) In pursuit of the study of pleasure: Implications for health research and practice. *Health: An Interdisciplinary Journal for the Social Study of Health, Illness and Medicine* 7(2): 161–79.

Crabbe, T. (2013) *Sportworks: Investing in sport for development – creating the business case to help change the lives of disadvantaged young people in the UK.* Manchester, England: Substance.

Crabbe, T. (2008) Avoiding the numbers game: Social theory, policy and sport's role in the art of relationship building. In M. Nicholson and R. Hoye (eds) *Sport and social capital.* London: Elsevier, pp. 21–37.

Crabbe, T. (2000) A sporting chance? Using sport to tackle drug use and crime. *Drugs: Education, Prevention and Policy* 7: 381–91.

Crawford, G. (2004) *Consuming sport: Fans, sport and culture.* London: Routledge.

Crichter, C. (2011) For a political economy of moral panics. *Crime, Media, Culture* 7(3): 259–75.

Crocket, H. (2014) An ethic of indulgence? Alcohol, Ultimate Frisbee and calculated hedonism. *International Review for the Sociology of Sport.* doi:10.1177/1012690214543960.

Crocket, H. (2013) 'This is *men's* ultimate': (Re)creating multiple masculinities in elite open Ultimate Frisbee. *International Review for the Sociology of Sport* 48(3): 318–33.

Crundall, I. (2012) Alcohol management in community sports clubs: Impact on viability and participation. *Health Promotion Journal of Australia* 23(2): 97–100.

Cunningham, J. and Beneforti, M. (2005) Investigating indicators for measuring the health and social impact of sport and recreation programs in Australian Indigenous communities. *International Review for the Sociology of Sport* 40(1): 89–98.

Curi, M., Knijnik, J. and Mascarenhas, G. (2011) The Pan American Games in Rio de Janeiro 2007: Consequences of a sport mega-event on a BRIC country. *International Review for the Sociology of Sport* 46(2): 140–56.

Curry, T.J. (2000) Booze and bar fights: A journey to the dark side of college athletics. In J. McKay, M.A. Messner and D. Sabo (eds) *Masculinities, gender relations and sport.* Thousand Oaks, CA: Sage, pp. 162–75.

Curry, T.J. (1998) Beyond the locker room: Campus bars and college athletes. *Sociology of Sport Journal* 15: 205–15.

Daly, J. (2006) *My life in and out of the rough.* London: !T Books.

Darnell, S. (2010) Power, politics and 'sport for development and peace': Investigating the utility of sport for international development. *Sociology of Sport Journal* 27(1): 54–75.

Davidson, J. and Bondi, L. (2004) Spatialising affect, Affecting space: Introducing emotional geographies. *Gender, Place and Culture* 11(3): 373–4.

Day, K., Gough, B. and McFadden, M. (2004) Warning! Alcohol can seriously damage your feminine health: A discourse analysis of recent British newspaper coverage of women and drinking. *Feminist Media Studies* 4: 165–83.

Dean, M. (1994) *Governmentality: Power and rule in modern society*. London: Sage.

de Garine, I. and de Garine, V. (eds) (2002) *Drinking: Anthropological approaches*. New York: Berghan Books.

Demant, J. (2009) When alcohol acts: An actor-network approach to teenagers, alcohol and parties. *Body & Society* 15(1): 25–46.

Demant, J. and Bruvik-Heinskou, M. (2011) Taking a chance: Sex, alcohol and acquaintance rape. *Young. Nordic Journal of Youth Studies* 19(4): 397–415.

Demetriou, D. (2005) Connell's concept of hegemonic masculinity: A critique. *Theory and Society* 30(3): 337–361.

Dempster, S. (2011) I drink, therefore I'm man: Gender discourses, alcohol and the construction of British undergraduate masculinities. *Gender and Education* 23(5): 635–53.

Department of Health (2010) *Annual Report of the Chief of Medical Officer*. London: Department of Health.

De Visser, R. and McDonnell, E. (2012) 'That's ok. He's a guy': A mixed-methods study of gender double-standards for alcohol use. *Psychology and Health* 27(5): 618–39.

Dewalt, K. Dewalt, B., with Wayland, C.B. (1998) Participant observation. In H.R. Bernard (ed.) *Handbook of methods in cultural anthropology*. Walnut Creek, CA: Alta Mira Press, pp. 259–99.

Dimeo, P. (2013). *Drugs, alcohol and sport: A critical history*. London: Routledge.

Dimovski, T., and Paunova, D. (2012) The impact of the 'Choose Life, Choose Sports' social campaign of the Agency of Youth and Sports on the healthy lifestyle promotion. *Activities In Physical Education & Sport* 2(2): 228–30.

Dixon, K. (2014) The football fan and the pub: An enduring relationship. *International Review for the Sociology of Sport* 49(3/4): 382–99.

Dixon, K. (2011) A 'third way' for football fandom research: Anthony Giddens and structuration theory. *Soccer and Society* 12(2): 279–98.

Dobson, S. Brudalen, R. and Tobiasson H. (2006) Courting risk – The attempt to understand youth cultures. *Young. Nordic Journal of Youth Studies* 1: 49–58.

Donnelly, M. (2013) Drinking with the derby girls: Exploring the hidden ethnography in research of women's flat track roller derby. *International Review for the Sociology of Sport* 49(3–4): 464–84.

Douglas, M. (1992) *Risk and blame: Essays in cultural theory*. London and New York: Routledge.

Douglas, M. (ed.) (1987) *Constructive drinking: Perspectives on drink from anthropology*. Cambridge: Cambridge University Press.

Douglas, M. (1966) *Purity and danger: An analysis of concepts of pollution and taboo*. New York: Praeger.

Douglas, M. and Wildavsky, A. (1982) *Risk and culture: An essay on the selection of technical and environmental dangers*. Berkeley: University of California Press.

Duff, C. (2008) Pleasure in context. *International Journal of Drug Policy* 19(5): 384–92.

Duff, C. and Munro, G. (2007) Preventing alcohol-related problems in community sports clubs: The Good Sports Program. *Substance Use & Misuse* 42(12/13): 1991–2001.

Du Gay, P. (1997) *Production of culture/Cultures of production.* London: Sage.

Dun, S. (2014) No beer, no way! Football fan identity enactment won't mix with Muslim beliefs in the Qatar 2022 World Cup. *Journal of Policy Research in Tourism, Leisure and Events* 6(2): 186–99.

Dunning, E. and Waddington, I. (2003) Sport as a drug and drugs in sport. *International Review for the Sociology of Sport* 38(3): 351–68.

Durant, R. and Thakker, J. (2003) *Substance use and abuse: Cultural and historical Perspectives.* London: Sage.

Dwyer, R. (2008) Privileging pleasures: Temazepam injection in a heroin marketplace. *International Journal of Drug Policy* 19(5): 367–74.

Elmeland, K and Kolind, T. (2012) 'Why don't they just do what we tell them?' Different alcohol prevention discourses in Denmark. *Young. Nordic Journal of Youth Studies* 20(2): 177–97.

Esenbach-Stangl, I. and Thom, B. (2009) Intoxication and intoxicated behaviour in contemporary European cultures: Myths, realities and the implications for policy, (prevention) practice and research.

Ewen, S. (1973) *Captains of consciousness: Advertising and the social roots of consumer culture.* New York: McGraw Hill.

Featherstone, M. (1994) *Consumer culture and postmodernism.* London: Sage.

Fenwick, M. and Hayward, K.J. (2000) Youth crime, excitement and consumer culture: The reconstruction of aetiology in contemporary criminological theory. In J. Pickford (ed.) *Youth Justice: Theory and Practice.* London: Cavendish.

Fletcher, T. and Spracklen, K. (2013) Cricket, drinking and exclusion of British Pakistani Muslims. *Ethnic and Racial Studies*: 1–19.

Flood, M. (2008) Men, sex and homo-sociality: How bonds between men shape their sexual relations with women. *Men and Masculinities* 10: 339–59.

Flood, M. (2002) Between men and masculinity: An assessment of the 'term' masculinity in recent scholarship on men. In S. Pearce and V. Muller (eds) *Manning the next millennium: Studies in masculinities.* Perth: Black Swan, pp. 203–13.

Ford, J. (2007) Alcohol use among college students: A comparison of athletes and non-athletes. *Substance Use and Abuse* 42(9): 1367–77.

Foucault, M. (1991) Governmentality. In G. Burchell, C. Gordon and P. Miller (eds) *The Foucault effect.* Chicago: University of Chicago Press, pp. 87–104.

Foucault, M. (1988) *Technologies of the self.* Minneapolis: University of Massachusetts Press.

Frank, A. (1991) *At the will of the body: Reflections on illness.* New York, NY: Houghton Mifflin Co.

Fuchs, J. and Le Hénaff, Y. (2013) Alcohol consumption among women rugby players in France: Uses of the 'third half time'. *International Review for the Sociology of Sport* 49(3–4): 434–46.

Gadd, D. (2006) The role of recognition in the desistance process: A case analysis of a former far-right activist. *Theoretical Criminology* 10(2): 179–202.

Gadd, D. and Farrall, S. (2004) Criminal careers, desistance and subjectivity interpreting men's narratives of change. *Theoretical Criminology* 8(2): 123–56.

Gamson, W.A. (1989) News as framing. *American Behavioral Scientist* 33(2): 157–61.

Gee, S., Jackson, S. and Sam, M. (2014) Carnivalesque culture and alcohol promotion and consumption at an annual international sports event in New Zealand. *International Review for the Sociology of Sport* 49(2). doi:10.1177/1012690214522461.

Gee, S. (2013) The culture of alcohol sponsorship during the 2011 Rugby World Cup: An (auto)ethnographic and (con)textual analysis. *Sport in Society* 16(7): 912–30.

Gilbert, M.J. (1993) Anthropology in a multidisciplinary field: Substance abuse. *Social Science and Medicine* 37(1): 1–3.

Gill, J.S. (2002) Reported levels of alcohol consumption and binge drinking within the UK undergraduate student population over the last 25 years. *Alcohol & Alcoholism* 37: 109–20.

Gitlin, T. (1980) *The whole world is watching: Mass media in the making and unmaking of the left.* Berkeley, CA: University of California.

Giuliannotti, R. (2004) Human rights, globalization and sentimental education: The case of sport. *Sport in Society* 7: 355–69.

Giulianotti, R. (1995) Football and the politics of carnival: An ethnographic study of Scottish football fans in Sweden. *International Review for the Sociology of Sport* 30: 191–217.

Gjernes, T. (2010) Facing resistance to health advice. *Health, Risk & Society* 12(5): 471–89.

Glassman, T.J., Dodd, V.J., Sheu, J.J., Rienzo, B.A. and Wagenaar, A.C. (2010) Extreme ritualistic alcohol consumption among college students on game day. *Journal of American College Health* 58(5): 413–23.

Glasner, P. (1977) *The sociology of secularization: A critique of a concept.* London: Routledge & Kegan Paul.

Goffman, E. (1959) *The presentation of self in everyday life.* New York: Doubleday.

Gogarty, P. and Williamson, I. (2009) *Winning at all costs: Sporting Gods and their demons.* London: JR Books.

Gordon, R., Hein, D. and MacAskill, S. (2012) Rethinking drinking cultures: A review of drinking cultures and a reconstructed dimensional approach. *Public Health* 126: 3–11.

Gorgulho, M. and Da Ros, V. (2006) Alcohol and harm reduction in Brazil. *International Journal of Drug Policy* 17: 350–57.

Gough, B. and Edwards, G. (1988) The beer talking: Four lads, a carry out and the reproduction of masculinities. *The Sociological Review* 46(3): 409–35.

Granfield, R. and Cloud, W. (2001) Social context and natural recovery: The role of social capital in the resolution of drug-associated problems. *Substance Use & Misuse* 36: 1543–70.

Granskog, J. (1992) Tri-ing together: an exploratory analysis of the social network of female and male triathletes. *Play & Culture* 5(1): 76–91.

Gratton, C. and Henry, I. (2001) *Sport and the city: The role of sport in economic and social generation.* London: Routledge.

Griffin, C. and Bengry-Howell, A., Hackley, C., Mistral, W. and Szmigin, I. (2009) 'Every time I do it, I absolutely annihilate myself': loss of (self) consciousness and loss of memory in young people's drinking narratives. *Sociology* 43(3): 457–76.

Griggs, G. (2011) 'This must be the only sport in the world where most of the players don't know the rules': Operationalizing self-refereeing and the spirit of the game in UK Ultimate Frisbee. *Sport in Society* 14(1): 97–110.

Groshkova, T. and Best, D. (2011) The evolution of a UK evidence base for substance misuse recovery. *Journal of Groups in Addiction & Recovery* 6(1): 20–37.

Guardian (2014) Torah Bright: Sochi poster girl or rebellious outsider? Available at: <http://www.theguardian.com/sport/blog/2014/feb/17/torah-bright-sochi-poster-girl-or-rebellious-outsider/print> (accessed 10 May 2015).

Gurney, J.N. (1985) Not one of the guys: The female researcher in a male-dominated setting. *Qualitative Sociology* 8(1): 42–62.

Gurney, J.N. (1991) Female researchers in male dominated settings. In W.B Shaffir and R.A Stebbins (eds) *Experiencing fieldwork: An inside view of qualitative research.* London: Sage, pp. 53–61.

Hackley, C., Bengry-Howell, A., Griffin, C., Mistral, W., Szmigin, I. and Hackley, R.A (2012). Young adults and 'binge' drinking: A Bakhtinian analysis. *Journal of Marketing Management*, Online First.

Hacking, I. (1986) 'Making up people'. In T.C. Heller (ed.) *Reconstructing individualism: Autonomy, individuality and the self in western thought.* Stanford, CA: Stanford University Press, pp. 222–36.

Hall, S. and Jefferson, T. (eds) *Resistance through rituals: Youth subcultures in post-war Britain.* London: Harper Collins.

Hamilton, C. (1994) *Absolut.* New York and London: Texerre.

Hannerz, U. (1989) Notes on the global ecumene. *Public Culture* 1: 66–75.

Hargreaves, J. (2007) Sport, exercise, and the female Muslim body: Negotiating Islam, politics, and male power. In J. Hargreaves and P. Vertinsky (eds) *Physical culture, power, and the body.* London and New York: Routledge, pp. 74–100.

Harrison, L., et al. (2011) 'I don't know anyone that has two drinks a day': Young people, alcohol and the government of pleasure. *Health, Risk & Society* 13(5): 469–86.

Harrison, L. (2008) 'I don't really care about what someone else's studied': Drinking guidelines and the government of pleasure. In T. Majoribanks, J. Barraket, J.-S. Chang, A. Dawson, M. Guillemin, M. Henry-Waring, A. Kenyon, R. Kokanovic, J. Lewis, D. Lusher, D. Nolan, P. Pyett, R. Robins,

D. Warr and J. Wyn (eds) *TASA 2008 : Re-imagining sociology : The annual conference of the Australian Sociological Association 2008, 2–5 December 2008, The University of Melbourne*, pp. 1–14, TASA, Melbourne, Vic.

Hartman, D. and Kwauk, C. (2011) Sport and development: An overview, critique and reconstruction. *Journal of Sport and Social Issues* 25: 339–71.

Haudenyhuyse, R. Theebom, M. and Nols, Z. (2012) Sports-based interventions for socially vulnerable youth: Towards well-defined interventions with easy-to-follow outcomes. *International Review for the Sociology of Sport* 48(4): 471–84.

Hawkins, B., Holden, C. and McCambridge, J. (2012) Alcohol industry influence on UK alcohol policy: A new research agenda for public health. *Critical Public Health* 22(3): 297–305.

Hayward, K. and Hobbs, D. (2003) Beyond the binge in 'booze Britain': Market-led liminalization and the spectacle of binge drinking. *The British Journal of Sociology* 58(3): 437–56.

Health. D. (2000) *Drinking occasions: Comparative perspectives on alcohol and culture.* International Centre for Alcohol Policies Series on Alcohol in Society. Philadelphia: Taylor and Francis.

Heath, D.B. (ed.) (1995) *International handbook on alcohol and culture.* Westport, CT: Greenwood Press.

Hellision, D. (2003) *Teaching responsibility through physical activity.* (2nd edn) Champaign, Il: Human Kinetics.

Hennessey, J. (2000) *Eye of the Hurricane: The Alex Higgins Story.* London: Mainstream Publishing.

Herman-Kinney, N. and Kinney, D. (2012) Sober as deviant: The stigma of sobriety and how some college students 'stay dry' on a 'wet' campus. *Journal of Contemporary Ethnography*: 1–40.

Heyes, C.J. (2006) Foucault goes to Weight Watchers. *Hypatia* 21(2): 126–49.

Higuchi, S., Matsushita, S. and Osaki, Y. (2006) Drinking practices, alcohol policy and prevention programs in Japan. *International Journal of Drug Policy* 17: 358–66.

Hobbs, D., Hadfield, P., Lister, S. and Winlow, S. (2003) *Bouncers: Violence and governance in the night-time economy.* Oxford: Oxford University Press.

Holder, H.D. (2004) Community action from an international perspective. In R. Muller and H. Klingemann (eds) *From science to action? 100 years later – alcohol policies revisited.* Dordecht, Netherlands: Kluwer Academic.

Holder, H.D. (2000) Community prevention of alcohol problems. *Addictive Behaviours* 25: 843–59.

Holloway, S., Jayne, M. and Valentine, G. (2008) 'Sainsbury's is my local': English alcohol policy, domestic drinking practices and the meaning of home. *Transactions. Journal of the Institute of British Geographers* 33(4): 532–47.

Holmila, M. and Raitasalo, K. (2005) Gender differences in drinking: why do they still exist? *Addiction* 100(12): 1763–9.

Holt, R. (1990) *Sport and the British: A modern history.* Oxford: Clarendon Press.

Honkassalo, M. (1989) 'Have the wives over for a sauna when I go out with the men!' In E. Haavio-Manila (ed.) *Women, alcohol and drugs in the Nordic countries* 16. Helsinki: Nordic Council for Alcohol and Drug Research.

Horne, J. and Whannel, G. (2009). Beer sponsors football: what could go wrong? In L. Wenner and S. Jackson (eds) *Sport, beer, and gender in promotional culture: Explorations of a holy trinity.* New York: Peter Lang, pp. 55–74.

Houlihan, B. (1994) Homogenisation, Americanization and creolization of sport: Varieties of globalization. *Sociology of Sport Journal* 11: 356–75.

Hunt, G., Mackenzie, K. and Joe-Laidler, K. (2005) Alcohol and masculinity: the case of ethnic youth gangs. In T.W. Wilson (ed.) *Drinking cultures: Alcohol and identity.* Oxford: Berg.

Hunt, G. and Barker, J. (2001) Socio-cultural anthropology and alcohol and drug research: towards a unified theory. *Social Science & Medicine* 53: 165–88.

Hutton, F. (2012) Harm reduction, students and pleasure: An examination of student responses to a binge drinking campaign. *International Journal of Drug Policy* 23: 229–35.

Hutton, F. (2004) *Risky pleasures: Club cultures and feminine identities.* Aldershot: Ashgate.

Hser, Y., Longshore, D. and Anglin, M. (2007) The life course perspective on drug use: A conceptual framework for understanding drug use trajectories. *Evaluation Review* 31: 515–47.

Jacobsen, G. (2003). Alcohol ads wet whistle of youth sport clubs. *The Sydney Morning Herald.*

Jackson, C. and Tinkler, P. (2007) 'Ladettes' and 'modern girls': 'Troublesome' young femininities. *The Sociological Review* 55(2): 251–72.

Jackson, S., Andrews, D. and Scherer, J. (2005) The commercial landscape of sport advertising. In S. Jackson, D. Andrews and J. Scherer (eds) *Sport, culture and advertising: Identities, commodities and the politics of representation.* London: Routledge.

Järvinen, M. and Østergaard, J. (2011) Dangers and pleasures: Drug attitudes and experiences among young people. *Acta Sociolgoica* 54 (4): 333–50.

Jaunin, R. (2007) *Roger Federer: Number One.* Lausanne: Editions Favre.

Jawad, H., Al-Sinani, Y. and Benn, T. (2011) Islam, women and sport. In T. Benn, G. Pfister and J. Jawad (eds) *Muslim women and sport.* London and New York: Routledge, pp. 25–40.

Jayne, M., Gibson, C., Waitt, G. and Valentine, G. (2012) Drunken mobilities: Backpackers, alcohol, 'doing place'. *Tourist Studies* 12(3): 211–31.

Jayne, M., Valentine, G. and Holloway S.L. (2008a) Geographies of alcohol, drinking and drunkenness: A review of progress. *Progress in Human Geography* 32: 243–59.

Jayne, M., Valentine, G. and Holloway S.L. (2008b) The place of drink: Geographical contributions to alcohol studies. *Drugs: Education, Prevention and Policy* 15: 219–32.

Jayne, M., Holloway, S.L. and Valentine, G. (2006) Drunk and disorderly: Alcohol, urban life and public space. *Progress in Human Geography* 30(4): 451–68.

Jones, C. (2014) Alcoholism and recovery: A case study of a former professional footballer. *International Review for the Sociology of Sport* 49: 485–505.

Jones, R.L. (2006) Dilemmas, maintaining 'face' and paranoia: An average coaching life. *Qualitative Inquiry* 12(5): 1012–21.

Jones, S.C., Phillipson, L. and Lynch, M. (2006) Alcohol and sport: Can we have one without the other? In *Faculty of Health & Behavioural Sciences – Papers.* University of Wollongong.

Keane, H. (2013) Healthy adults and maternal bodies: Reformulations of gender in Australian alcohol guidelines. *Health Sociology Review* 22(2): 151–61.

Keane, H. (2009) Foucault on methadone: Beyond biopower. *International Journal of Drug Policy* 20: 450–52.

Kelly, L. (2012) Sports-based interventions and the local governance of youth crime and anti-social behaviour. *Journal of Sport & Social Issues* 37(3): 261–83.

Kelly, L. (2011). 'Social inclusion' through sports-based interventions? *Critical Social Policy* 31(1): 126–50.

Kelly, P., Hickey, C., Cormack., S. Harrison, L. and Lindsay, J. (2011) Charismatic cops, patriarchs and a few good women: Leadership culture and young people's drinking. *Sport, Education and Society* 16(4): 467–84.

Kelly, B., King, L., Bauman, A.E., Baur, L.A., Macniven, R., Chapman, K. and Smith, B.J. (2014) Identifying important and feasible policies and actions for health at community sports clubs: A consensus-generating approach. *Journal of Science and Medicine in Sport* 17(1): 61–6.

Killingworth, B. (2006) Drinking stories from a playgroup: Alcohol in the lives of middle class mothers in Australia. *Ethnography* 7(3): 357–84.

King, A. (1997) The lads: Masculinity and the new consumption of football. *Sociology* 31(2): 329–46.

Kingsland, M., Wolfenden, L., Rowland, B.C., Gillham, K.E., Kennedy, V.J., Ramsden, R.L., Colbran, R.W., Weir, S. and Wiggers, J.H. (2013) Alcohol consumption and sport: A cross-sectional study of alcohol management practices associated with at-risk alcohol consumption at community football clubs. *BMC Public Health* 13: 1–9.

Kraszewski, J. (2008) Pittsburgh in Fort Worth: Football bars, sports television, sport fandom and the management of home. *Journal of Sport & Social Issues* 32(2): 139–57.

Lake, R. (2012) 'They treat me like I'm scum': Social exclusion and established-outsider relations in a British tennis club. *International Review for the Sociology of Sport* 48(1): 112–28.

Landale, S. and Roderick, M. (2013) Recovery from addiction and the potential role of sport: Using a life course theory to study change. *International Review for the Sociology of Sport* 49(3–4): 377–93.

Landale, S. (2012) *Transitions and turning points: Efficacy of sport-based drugs intervention programs in desistance.* Unpublished PhD Thesis, School of Social Sciences, Durham University, UK.

Laub, J. and Sampson, R. (2003) *Shared beginnings, divergent lives: Delinquent boys to Age 70.* Cambridge, MA: Harvard University Press.

Laurendau, J. (2008) Gendered risk regimes: a theoretical consideration of edgework and gender. *Sociology of Sport* 25(3): 293–309.

Leaver-Dunn, D., Turner, L. and Newman, B. (2007) Influence of sports' programs and club activities on alcohol use intentions and behaviors among adolescent males. *Journal of Alcohol & Drug Education* 51(3): 57–72.

Le Breton, D. (2000) Playing symbolically with death in extreme sports. *Body & Society* 6(1): 1–11.

Leskelä-Kärki, M. (2008) Narrating life stories in between the fictional and the autobiographical. *Qualitative Research* 8(3): 325–32.

Levi, R. and Valverde, M. (2001) Knowledge on tap: Police science and common knowledge in the legal regulation of drunkenness. *Law & Social Inquiry* 26: 819–46.

Leyshon, M. (2005) No place for a girl. Rural youth, pubs and the performance of masculinity. In J. Little and C. Morris (eds) *Critical studies in rural gender issues.* Aldershot: Ashgate.

Lindsay, J. (2010) Health living guidelines and the disconnect with everyday life. *Critical Public Health* 20(4): 475–87.

Lindsay, J. (2009) Young Australians and the staging of intoxication and self-control. *Journal of Youth Studies* 12(4): 371–84.

Lindsay, J. (2006) A big night out in Melbourne: Drinking as an enactment of class and gender. *Contemporary Drug Problems* 33(1): 29–61.

Lines, G. (2001) Villains, fools or heroes? Sports stars as role models for young people. *Leisure Studies* 20(4): 285–303.

Lipsky, M. (1980) *Street level bureaucracy.* London: Sage.

Litchfield, C. and Dionigi, R.A. (2012) Rituals in Australian women's veteran's field hockey. *International Journal of Sport & Society* 3(3): 171–85.

Lhussier, M. and Carr, S.M. (2008) Health related lifestyle advice: critical insights. *Critical Public Health* 18 (3): 299–309.

Lock, C.A. (2004) Alcohol and brief intervention in primary health care: What do patients think? *Primary Health Care Research and Development* 5: 162–78.

Lucas, N., Windsor, T., Caldwell, T. and Rodgers, B. (2010) Psychological distress in non-drinkers: Associations with previous heavy drinking and current social relationships. *Alcohol and Alcoholism* 45(1): 95–102.

Lunnay, B., Ward, P. and Borlagdan, J. (2011) The practice and practice of Bourdieu: The application of social theory to youth alcohol research. *International Journal of Drug Policy* 22: 428–36.

Lupton, D. (1999) *Risk.* London: Routledge.

Lupton, D. (1995) *The imperative of health: Public health and the regulated body.* London: Sage.

Lupton, D. and Tulloch, J. (2002) 'Life would be pretty dull without risk': Voluntary risk-taking and its pleasures. *Health, Risk & Society* 4: 113–24.

Lyng, S. (2005) *Edgework: The sociology of risk-taking*. London: Routledge.

Lyng, S. (1990) Edgework: A social psychological analysis of voluntary risk taking. *American Journal of Sociology* 95(4): 851–86.

Lyons, A. and Willott, S. (2008) Alcohol consumption, gender identities and women's changing social positions. *Sex Roles* 59: 694–712.

Lyons, K. (1991) Telling stories from the field? A discussion of an ethnographic approach to researching the teaching of physical education. In A. Sparkes (ed.) *Research in physical education and sport – Exploring alternative visions.* London: Falmer Press, pp. 248–70.

MacAndrew, C. and Edgerton, R. (1969) *Drunken comportment: A social explanation.* Chicago: Aldine.

McCreanor, T., Lyons, A., Griffin, C., Goodwin, I., Moewaka Barnes, H. and Hutton, F. (2013) Youth drinking cultures, social networking and alcohol marketing: Implications for public health. *Critical Public Health* 23(1): 110–20.

McDonald, M. (ed.) (1994) *Gender, drink and drugs*. Oxford: Berg Publishers.

McDonald, B. and Sylvester, K. (2013) Learning to get drunk: The importance of drinking in Japanese university sports clubs. *International Review for the Sociology of Sport*: 1–15.

McKay, J., Messner, M. and Sabo, D. (eds) (2000). *Studying sport from feminist standpoints.* London: Sage.

McIntosh, J. and McKeganey, N. (2002) *Beating the dragon: The recovery from dependent drug use.* Harlow: Prentice Hall.

Maclennan, B., Kypri, K., Langley, J. and Room, R. (2012) Public sentiment towards alcohol and local government alcohol policies in New Zealand. *International Journal of Drug Policy* 23: 45–53.

McRobbie, A. (1994) *Postmodernism and Popular Culture*: London. Routledge.

McCreanor, T, Lyons, A., Griffin, C., et al. (2013) Youth drinking cultures, social networking and alcohol marketing: Implications for public health. *Critical Public Health* 23(1): 110–20.

Magee, J. and Jeans, R. (2011) Football's coming home: A critical evaluation of the Homeless World Cup as an intervention to combat social exclusion. *International Review for the Sociology of Sport* 48(1): 3–19.

Maggs, J., Rankin, L. and Lee, C. (2011) Ups and downs of alcohol use among First-year college students: Number of drinks, heavy drinking, and stumble and pass out drinking days. *Addictive Behaviours* 36(3): 197–202.

Mansfield, L. and Rich, E. (2013) Public health pedagogy, border crossings and physical activity at very size. *Critical Public Health* 23(3): 356–70.

Markula, P. (2009) Acceptable bodies: Deconstructing the Finish media coverage of the 2004 Olympic Games. In P. Markula (ed.) *Olympic women and the media: International perspectives*. New York: Palgrave Macmillan, pp. 87–111.

Markula, P. (2004) 'Turning into one's self': Foucault's technologies of the self and mindful fitness. *Sociology of Sport Journal* 21(3): 302–21.

Markula, P. (2003) The technologies of the self: Sport, feminism, and Foucault. *Sociology of Sport Journal* 20: 87–107.

Martin, M. (2012) The impossible sexual difference: Representations from a rugby union setting. *International Review for the Sociology of Sport* 47(2): 183–99.

Measham, F. (2006) The new policy mix: alcohol, harm minimisation and determined drunkenness in contemporary society. *International Journal of Drug Policy* 17(4): 258–68.

Measham, F. (2004a) The decline of ecstasy, the rise of 'binge drinking' and the persistence of pleasure. *Probation Journal* 5(4): 309–26.

Measham, F. (2004b) Play space: Historical and socio-cultural reflections on drugs, licensed leisure locations, commercialisation and control. *International Journal of Drug Policy* 15: 337–45.

Measham, F. (2003) The gendering of drug use and the absence of gender. *Criminal Justice Matters* 53(1): 22–3.

Measham, F. (2002) Doing gender – doing drugs. Conceptualising the gendering of drug cultures. *Contemporary Drug Problems* 29(2).

Measham, F. and Østergaard, J. (2009) The public face of binge drinking: British and Danish young women, recent trends in alcohol consumption and the European binge drinking debate. *Probation Journal* 56(4): 415–34.

Measham, F. and Shiner, M. (2009) The legacy of 'normalization': The role of classical and contemporary criminological theory in understanding young people's drug use. *International Journal of Drug Policy* 20: 502–8.

Measham, F. and Brain, K. (2005) 'Binge' drinking, British alcohol policy and the new culture of intoxication. *Crime, Media Culture* 1(3): 262–83.

Measham, F., Aldridge, J. and Parker, H. (2001) *Dancing on drugs: Risk, health and hedonism in the British club scene*. London: Free Association Books.

Meek, R. and Lewis, G. (2012) The role of sport in promoting prisoner health. *International Journal of Prisoner Health* 8(3/4): 117–30.

Messerschmidt, J.W. (1995) From patriarchy to gender: Feminist theory, criminology, and the challenge of diversity. In N. Hahn Rafter and F. Heidensohn (eds) *International Feminist perspectives in Criminology*. Philadelphia: Open University Press, pp. 167–88.

Mewett, P. and Toffoletti, K. (2011) Finding footy: Female fan socialization and Australian rules football. *Sport in Society* 14(5): 670–84.

Mills, C. Wright ([1959] 2000) *The sociological imagination*. Oxford: Oxford University Press.

Millward, P. (2009) Glasgow Rangers supporters in the city of Manchester: The degeneration of a 'fan party' into a 'hooligan riot'. *International Review for the Sociology of Sport* 44(4): 381–98.

Mistral, W., Vellerman, R., Templeton, L. and Mastache, C. (2006) Local action to prevent alcohol problems: Is the UK community alcohol prevention programme the best solutions? *International Journal of Drug Policy* 17: 278–84.

Moore, D. (2008) Erasing pleasure from public discourse on illicit drugs: On the creation and reproduction of an absence. *International Journal of Drug Policy* 19(5): 353–8.

Moore, D. (2002) Ethnography and the Australian drug field: Emancipation, appropriation and multidisciplinarity in the drug field. *International Journal of Drug Policy* 13(4).

Moore, D. (1992) Penetrating social worlds: Conducting ethnographic research on drug and alcohol use in Australia. *Drug and Alcohol Review* 11: 313–23.

Moore, D. (1990) Drinking, the construction of ethnic identity, and social process in a Western Australian youth subculture. *British Journal of Addiction* 84: 1265–78.

Moore, D. and Maher, L. (eds) (2002) Special issue: Ethnography and multidisciplinarity in the drug field. *International Journal of Drug Policy* 13(4).

Moore, D. and Rhodes, T. (2004) Social theory in drug research, drug policy and harm reduction. *International Journal of Drug Policy* 15(5): 323–5.

Morris, L., Sallybanks, J. and Willis, K. (2003) *Sport, physical activity and anti-social behaviour in youth.* (No. 49). Canberra, Australian Institute of Criminology.

Morse, S.J. (2011) Addiction and criminal responsibility. In J. Poland and G. Graham (eds) *Addiction and responsibility.* Cambridge, MA: The MIT Press, pp. 159–20.

Muir, K.B. and Seitz, T. (2004) Machismo, misogyny, and homophobia in a male athletic subculture: A participant-observation study of deviant rituals in collegiate rugby. *Deviant Behavior* 25(4): 303–27.

Mullen, K., Watson, J., Swift, J., and Black, D. (2007) Young men, masculinity and alcohol. *Drugs-Education Prevention and Policy* 14: 151–65.

Mythen, G. (2004) *Ulrich Beck: A critical introduction to the risk society.* London: Pluto Press.

National Health and Medical Research Council (2001) *Australian alcohol guidelines: Health risks and benefits.* Canberra: AusInfo. Available at: <http://www.health.gov.au/nhmrc/publications/pdf/ds9.pdf> (accessed 10 May 2015).

Neale, J., Bloor, M. and McKeganey, N. (2007) How do heroin users spend their spare time? *Drugs: Education, Prevention and Policy* 14: 231–46.

Neale, J., Allen, D. and Coombes, L. (2005) Qualitative research methods within the addictions. *Addiction* 100: 1593–684.

Neale, J. (1998) Drug users' views of drug service providers. *Health and Social Care in the Community* 6: 308–17.

Nettleton, S. (1997) Governing the risky self: How to become healthy wealthy and wise. In R. Bunton and A. Petersen (eds) *Foucault, health and medicine.* London: Routledge, pp. 207–22.

Nettleton, S., Neale, J. and Pickering, L. (2011) 'I don't think there's much of a rational mind in a drug addict when they are in the thick of it': Towards an embodied analysis of recovering heroin users. *Sociology of Health & Illness* 33: 341–55.

Newburn, T. and Shiner, M. (2001) *Teenage kicks? Young people and alcohol: A review of the literature.* York, UK: Joseph Rowntree Foundation / York Publishing Service.

Nicheter, M., Quintero., Nichter, M., et al. (2004) Qualitative research: Contributions to the study of drug use, drug abuse and drug user-related interventions. *Substance Use & Misuse* 39(10–12): 1907–69.

Nichols, G. (2007) *Sport and crime reduction: The role of sports in tacking youth crime*. London: Routledge.

Nichols, G. and Crow, I. (2004) Measuring the impact of crime reduction interventions involving sports activities for young people. *Howard Journal of Criminal Justice* 43(3): 267–83.

Nixon, H. (1996) The relationship of friendship networks, sport experiences and gender to expressed pain thresholds. *Sociology of Sport Journal* 13: 78–86.

Nixon, H. (1993) Social network analysis in sport; emphasising social structure in sport. *Sociology of Sport Journal* 10: 315–21.

Nygaard, P., Waiters, E.D., Grube, J.W. and Keefe, D. (2003) Why do they do it? A qualitative study of adolescent drinking and driving. *Substance Use and Misuse* 38: 835–63.

O'Brien, K.S., Ali, A., Cotter, J., O'Shea, R. and Stannard, S. (2007) Hazardous drinking in New Zealand sportspeople: level of sporting participation and drinking motives. *Alcohol Alcoholism* 42(4): 376–82.

O'Malley, P. and Valverde, M. (2004) Pleasure, freedom and drugs: The uses of pleasure in liberal governance of drug and alcohol consumption. *Sociology* 38(1): 25–42.

Palmer, C. (2013a) Sport and alcohol-who's missing? New directions for a sociology of sport-related drinking. *International Review for the Sociology of Sport* 49(3–4): 263–78.

Palmer, C. (2013b) Drinking like a guy? Women and sport-related drinking. *Journal of Gender Studies* 23(2): 1–13.

Palmer, C. (2013c) *Global sports policy*. London: Sage.

Palmer, C. (2011) Key themes and research agendas in the sport-alcohol nexus. *Journal of Sport & Social Issues* 35(2): 168–85.

Palmer, C. (2009a) Soccer and the politics of identity for young refugee women in South Australia. *Soccer and Society* 10(1): 27–38.

Palmer, C. (2009b) 'The Grog Squad': An ethnography of beer consumption at Australian Rules football matches. In L. Wenner and S. Jackson (eds) *Sport, Beer and Gender in Promotional Culture: Explorations of a Holy Trinity*. New York: Peter Langm, pp. 225–41.

Palmer, C. (2004) Death, danger and the selling of risk in adventure sports. In B. Wheaton (ed.) *Understanding lifestyle sport: Consumption, identity, difference*. London: Routledge, pp. 55–69.

Palmer, C. (2000) Spin doctors and sports brokers: researching elites in contemporary sport – a research note on the Tour de France. *International Review for the Sociology of Sport* 35(3): 385–98.

Palmer, C. (1996) *A life of its own: the social construction of the Tour de France*. Unpublished PhD Thesis. Department of Anthropology, University of Adelaide.

Palmer, C. and Thompson, K. (2010) Everyday risks and professional dilemmas; Fieldwork with alcohol-based (sporting) subcultures. *Qualitative Research* 10(4): 1–20.

Palmer, C. and Thompson, K. (2007) The paradoxes of football spectatorship: on field and on line expressions of social capital among the Grog Squad. *Sociology of Sport Journal* 24: 187–205.

Parker, A. and Weir, J. (2012) Sport, spirituality and Protestantism: A historical overview. *Theology* 115(4): 253–65.

Parker, H., Aldridge, J. and Measham, F. (1998) *Illegal leisure: The normalization of recreational drug use.* London: Routledge.

Parry, M. and Malcolm, D. (2004) England's Barmy Army: Commercialization, masculinity and nationalism. *International Review for the Sociology of Sport* 39(1): 75–94.

Pawson, R. (2006) *Evidence-Based policy: A realist perspective.* London: SAGE.

Pawson, R. and Tilley, I. (2004) Realist evaluation. In *Paper prepared for the British Cabinet Office.* Available at: <http://www.communitymatters.com.au/RE_chapter.pdf> (accessed 10 May 2015).

Peace, A. (1998) Anthropology in the postmodern landscape: the importance of cultural brokers and their trade. *The Australian Journal of Anthropology* 9(3): 274–85.

Peralta, R. and Jauk, D., (2011) A brief Feminist review and critique of the sociology of alcohol-use and substance-abuse treatment approaches. *Sociology Compass* 5(10): 882–97.

Peralta, R., Steele, J., Nofziger, S. and Rickles, M. (2010) The impact of gender on binge drinking behaviour among U.S college students attending a mid-western university: An analysis of two gender measures. *Feminist Criminology* 5(4): 355–79.

Peralta, R. and Steele, J. (2009) On drinking styles and race: A consideration of the socio-structural determinants of alcohol use and behaviour. *Journal of Ethnicity in Substance Abuse* 8(2): 146–62.

Peralta, R. (2007) College alcohol use and the embodiment of hegemonic masculinity among European American men. *Sex Roles* 56: 741–56.

Peterson, A., Davis, M., Fraser, S. and Lindsay, J (2010) Healthy living and citizenship: An overview. *Critical Public Health* 20(4): 391–400.

Pike, E. (2007) Revisiting the 'physical activity, sexual health, teenage identity construction' nexus. *International Review for the Sociology of Sport* 42(3): 309–19.

Plant, M., Plant, M. and Thornton, C. (2002) People and places: Some factors in the alcohol-violence link. *Journal of Substance Use* 7(4): 207–13.

Poland. J. and Graham, G. (2011) Introduction: The makings of a responsible addict. In: J. Poland and G. Graham (eds) *Addiction and responsibility.* Cambridge, MA: The MIT Press, pp. 1–19.

Popay, J., Bennett, S., Thomas, C., Williams, G., Gatrell, A. and Bostock, L. (2003) Beyond 'beer, fags, egg and chips'? Exploring lay understandings of social inequalities in health. *Sociology of Health & Illness* 25: 1–23.

Pope, S. (2011) 'Like pulling down Durham cathedral and building a brothel': women as 'new consumer' fans? *International Review for the Sociology of Sport* 46(4): 471–87.

Powers, J. and Young, A. (2008) Longitudinal analysis of alcohol consumption and health of middle-aged women in Australia. *Addiction* 103(3): 424–34.

President's Council on Physical Fitness and Sports (2006) *Sports and character development*. Research digest series 7(1). Washington, DC: President's Council on Physical Fitness and Sports.

Pringle, R. (2011) Masculinities, gender relations and leisure studies: Are we there yet? *Annals of Leisure Research* 14(2–3): 107–19.

Pringle, R. (2005) Masculinities, sport and power. *Journal of Sport and Social Issues* 29(3): 256–78.

Pringle, R. and Hickey, C. (2010). Negotiating masculinities via the moral problematization of sport. *Sociology of Sport Journal* 27(2): 115–39.

Ravenhill, M. (2008) *The culture of homelessness*. Aldershot: Ashgate.

Renker, P.R. (2003), Keeping safe: Teenagers' strategies for dealing with Perinatal Violence. *Journal of Obstetric, Gynecologic, & Neonatal Nursing* 32: 58–67.

Respect Task Force (2006) *Respect action plan*. London, UK: Home Office.

Reuters (2012) Heineken extends Rugby World Cup sponsorship for RWC 2015 in England. Available at: <http://www.reuters.com/article/2011/10/21/idUS65450+21-Oct-2011+HUG20111021> (accessed 10 May 2015).

Rhodes, T. (1995) Researching and theorizing 'risk': notes on the social relations of risk in heroin users' lifestyles. In P. Aggleton, G. Hart and P. Davies (eds) *AIDS: Sexuality, safety and risk*. London: Taylor & Francis, pp. 125–43.

Richards, D. (2012) Let fans drink. *London Evening Standard*, 14 March 2012. Available at: <www.standard.co.uk.pasportsfeeds/richards--letfansdrink_7567289.html> (accessed 10 May 2015).

Richardson, A. and Budd, T. (2003) Young adults, alcohol, crime and disorder. *Criminal Behaviour & Mental Health* 13(1): 6–16.

Robertson, S. (2003) 'If I let a goal in, I'll get beat up': Contradictions in masculinity, sport and health. *Health Education Research* 18(6): 706–16.

Roche, AM., Bywood, P. Borlagdan, J., Lunnay, B., Freeman, T., Lawton, L., Tovel, A. and Nicholas, R. (2007) *Young people & alcohol: the role of cultural influences, report*, National Centre for Education and Training on Addiction, Adelaide, p. 32.

Roche, M. (2003) Mega-events, time and modernity: On time structures in global society. *Time & Society* 12(1): 99–126.

Roche, M. (2000) *Mega-events and modernity: Olympics and Expos in the growth of global culture*. London: Routledge.

Roderick, M. (2006) *The work of professional football: A labour of love*. London: Routledge.

Rolando, S., Beccaria, F., Tigerstedt, C. and Torronen, J. (2012) First drink: What does it mean? The alcohol socialization process in different drinking cultures. *Drugs: Education, Prevention and Policy* 19(3): 201–12.

Room, R. (1996) Gender roles and interactions in drinking and drug use. *Journal of Substance Abuse* 8(2): 227–39.

Room, R. (1984) Alcohol and ethnography: A case of problem deflation? *Current Anthropology* 25(2): 169–91.

Room, R., Graham, K., Rehm, J., et al. (2003) Drinking and its burden in a global perspective: policy considerations and options. *European Addiction Research* 9: 165–75.

Rose, N. and Miller, P. (1992) Political power beyond the State: problematics of government. *British Journal of Sociology* 43(2): 173–205.

Rosen, M. (1988) You asked for it: Christmas at the bosses' expense. *Journal of Management Studies* 25(5): 463–80.

Rowland, B., Allen, F. and Toumbourou, J.W. (2012a) Association of risky alcohol consumption and accreditation in the 'Good Sports' alcohol management programme. *Journal of Epidemiology & Community Health* 66(8): 684–90.

Rowland, B., Allen, F. and Toumbourou, J.W. (2012b) Impact of alcohol harm reduction strategies in community sports clubs: Pilot evaluation of the Good Sports program. *Health psychology* 31(3): 323–33.

Rumbold, G. and Hamilton, M. (1998) Addressing drug problems: The case for harm minimisation. In M. Hamilton, A. Kellehear and G. Rumbold (eds) *Drug use in Australia: A harm minimisation approach.* Melbourne: Oxford University Press.

Sampson, R. and Laub, J. (2005) A life-course view of the development of crime. *Annals of the American Academy of Political and Social Science* 602: 12–44.

Sampson, H. and Thomas, M. (2003) Lone researchers at sea: Gender, risk and responsibility. *Qualitative Research* 3(2): 165–89.

Scherer, J. and Jackson, S. (2008) Producing Allblacks.com: Cultural intermediaries and the policing of electronic sporting consumption. *Sociology of Sport Journal* 25: 187–205.

Schaaf, P. (2005) Sports inc.: 100 years of sports business. Amehurst, NY: Prometheus Books.

Schuckit, M. and Smith, T. (2010) Onset and course of alcoholism over 25 years in middle class men. *Drug and Alcohol Dependence* 113(1): 21–8.

Schippers, V. (2007) Recovering the feminine other: masculinity, femininity, and gender hegemony. *Theory and Society* 36: 85–102.

Schwandt, T.A. (2001) *Dictionary of qualitative inquiry* (2nd ed.). Thousand Oaks, CA: Sage.

Scott, B. (2001) Beer. In R. Maxwell (ed.) *Culture works.* Minneapolis: University of Minnesota Press, pp. 60–82.

Scriven, M. (1994) The fine line between evaluation and explanation. *Evaluation Practice* 15: 75–7.

Seear, K. and Fraser, S. (2010) The 'sorry addict': Ben Cousins and the construction of drug use and addiction in elite sport. *Health Sociology Review* 19, Sociology, Recreational Drugs and Alcohol: 176–91.

Seddon, T. (2011) Explaining drug policy: Towards an historical sociology of policy change. *International Journal of Drug Policy* 22(6): 415–19.

Seidler, V. (2006) *Young men and masculinities: Global cultures and intimate lives*. New York: Zed Books.

Sherif, B. (2001) The ambiguity of boundaries in the fieldwork experience: Establishing rapport and negotiating insider/outsider status. *Qualitative Inquiry* 7(4): 437–47.

Sherry, E. (2010). (Re)engaging marginalised groups through sport development programs: the Homeless World Cup. *International Review for the Sociology of Sport* 45(1): 59–72.

Silverman, D. (2013) *Doing qualitative research: A practical handbook*. London: SAGE.

Singer, M. (1986) Towards a political economy of alcoholism: The missing link in the anthropology of drinking behaviour. *Social Science & Medicine* 23(2): 113–30.

Skeggs, B. (2005) The making of class and gender through visualizing moral subject formation. *Sociology* 39(5): 965–82.

Skeggs, B. (1997) *Formations of class and gender*. London: Sage.

Smith, K. (2012*) Kelly Smith footballer. My story*: London. Corgi Books.

Social Exclusion Unit (1998) *Bringing Britain Together*. London: Cabinet Office.

Spaaij, R. (2013) Cultural diversity in community sport: An ethnographic inquiry of Somali Australians' experiences. *Sport Management Review* 16(1): 29–40.

Spaaij, R. (2012) Building social and cultural capital among young people in disadvantaged communities: Lessons from a Brazilian sport-based intervention program. *Sport, Education and Society* 17(1): 77–95.

Spaaj, R. (2009) Sport as a vehicle for social mobility and regulation of disadvantaged urban youth. *International Review for the Sociology of Sport* 44: 247–64.

Spandler, H. and McKeown, M. (2012) A critical exploration of using football in health and welfare programs: Gender, masculinities, and social relations. *Journal of Sport and Social Issues* 36(4): 387–409.

Spracklen, K. (20013) Respectable drinkers, sensible drinkers, serious leisure: single malt whisky enthusiasts and the moral panic of irresponsible Others. *Contemporary Social Science: Journal of the Academy of Social Science* 8(1): 46–57.

Sparkes, A.C. (1996) 'The Fatal Flaw: A Narrative of the Fragile Body Self', *Qualitative Inquiry* 2: 463–94.

Sparkes, A.C. (1998) 'Narratives of Self as an Occasion of Conspiracy', *Sociology of Sport Online* 1(1) <http://physed.otago.ac.nz/sosol/v1i1/v1i1a3.htm> (accessed 10 August 2006).

Sparkes, A.C. (2002) *Telling tales in sport and physical activity: A qualitative journey.* Champaign, IL: Human Kinetics.

Stanko, E. (1999) Making the invisible visible in criminology: A personal Journey. In S. Holdaway and P. Rock (eds) *Thinking about Criminology.* London: UCL, pp. 35–54.

Stanley, L. (1992) *The auto/biographical I. The theory and practise of feminist auto/biography.* Manchester: Manchester University Press.

Stebbins, R.A. (2001) The costs and benefits of hedonism: Some consequences of taking casual leisure seriously. *Leisure Studies* 20(4): 305–9.

Stebbins, R.A. (1997) Casual leisure: A conceptual statement. *Leisure Studies* 16(1): 17–25.

Stebbins, R. (1992) *Amateurs, professionals and serious leisure.* Montreal and Kingston: McGill-Queens University Press.

Stevens, A. (2011) Editorial. Sociological approaches to the study of drug use and drug policy. *International Journal of Drug Policy* 22: 399–403.

Stewart, C., Smith, B. and Sparkes, A. (2011) Sporting autobiographies of illness and the role of metaphor. *Sport in Society* 9(5): 581–97.

Stranger, M. (2011) *Surfing life: Surface, substructure and the commodification of the sublime.* Farnham: Ashgate.

Sugden, J. and Tomlinson, A. (2011) Preface. In J. Sugden and A. Tomlinson (eds) *Watching the Olympics: Politics, power and representation.* London: Routledge.

Sugden, J. (1997) Field workers rush in (where theorists fear to tread): The perils of ethnography. In A. Tomlinson and S. Fleming (eds) *Ethics, Sport and Leisure: Crises and Critiques.* Toronto, ON, Canada: Meyer & Meyer Sport Ltd, pp. 223–44.

Szmigin, I., Griffin., and Mistral., W (2008) Reframing 'binge drinking' as 'calculated hedonism': Empirical evidence from the UK. *International Journal of Drug Policy* (19): 359–66.

Thompson, K., Palmer, C. and Raven, M. (2011) Drinkers, non-drinkers and deferrers: Reconsidering the beer/footy couplet amongst Australian Rules football fans. *The Australian Journal of Anthropology* 22(3): 388–408.

Thompson, L., Pearce, J. and Barnett, J. (2007) Moralising geographies: Stigma, smoking islands and responsible subjects. *Area* 39(4): 508–17.

Thornton, A. (2004) 'Anyone can play this game': Ultimate Frisbee, identity and difference. In B. Wheaton (ed.) *Understanding lifestyle sport: Consumption, identity and difference.* Oxon, UK: Routledge, pp. 175–96.

Thornton, S. (1995) *Club cultures: Music, media and subcultural capital.* Oxford: Polity.

Thorpe, H. (2012) Sex, drugs and snowboarding: (Il)legitimate definitions of taste and lifestyle in a physical youth culture. *Leisure Studies* 31(1): 35–51.

Thorpe, H. (2010) Bourdieu, gender reflexivity and physical culture. A case of masculinities in the snowboarding field. *Journal of Sport and Social Issues* 34(2): 176–214.

Thurnell-Read, T. (2012) 'Yobs' and 'snobs': Embodying drink and the problematic male body. *Sociological Research Online* 18(2/3).

Thurnell-Read, T. (2011a) Off the leash and out of control: Masculinities and embodiment in Eastern European stag tourism. *Sociology* 45(6): 977–91.

Thurnell-Read, T. (2011b) Here comes the drunken cavalry: Managing and negotiating the Britishness of all-male stag tours in Eastern Europe. In C. McGlynn, A. Mycock and J. McAuley (eds) *Britishness identity and citizenship: The view from abroad.* Berne: Peter Lang, pp. 215–31.

Tobin C.L., Fitzgerald, J.L., Livingstone, C., Thomson, I. and Harper, T.A. (2012) Support for breaking the nexus between alcohol and community sports settings: Findings from the VicHealth Community Attitudes Survey in Australia. *Drug & Alcohol Review* 31(4): 413–21.

Toffoletti, K. and Mewett, P. (eds) (2012) *Sport and its female fans.* London: Routledge.

Tonts, M. (2005) Competitive sport and social capital in rural Australia. *Journal of Rural Studies* 21: 137–49.

Tulle, E. (2014) Living by numbers: Media representations of sports stars' careers. *International Review for the Sociology of Sport*: 1–4.

Turner, V. (1967) *The Forest of Symbols*, Ithaca, NY: Cornell University Press.

Tutenges, S. (2009) Safety problems among heavy-drinking youth at a Bulgarian nightlife resort. *International Journal of Drug Policy* 20: 444–6.

Tutenges, S. and Rod, M.H. (2009) 'We got incredibly drunk … it was damned fun': Drinking stories among Danish youth. *Journal of Youth Studies* 12(4): 355–70.

Tutenges, S. and Sandberg, S. (2013). Intoxicating stories: The characteristics, contexts and implications of drinking stories among Danish youth. *International Journal of Drug Policy* 24: 538–44.

Vamplew, W. (1988) *Pay up and play the game: Professional sport in Britain 1875–1914.* Cambridge: Cambridge University Press.

Waitt, G. and Warren, A. (2008) 'Talking shit over a brew after a good session with your mates': Surfing, space and masculinity. *Australian Geographer* 39: 353–65.

Walsh, S. (2008) Helping youth in undeserved communities envision possible futures: An extension of the teaching personal and social responsibilities model. *Research Quarterly for Exercise and Sport* 79: 209–21.

Warren, C. (1988) Gender issues in field research. *Urban Life* 6(3): 349–69.

Weed, M. (2006) The story of an ethnography: The experience of watching the 2002 World Cup in the pub. *Soccer and Society* 7(1): 76–95.

Wenner, L. and Jackson, S. (2009) Sport, beer and gender in promotional culture: On the dynamics of the holy trinity. In L. Wenner and S. Jackson (eds) *Sport, beer, and gender in promotional culture: Explorations of a holy trinity.* New York: Peter Lang, pp. 1–34.

Wenner, L. (1991) One part alcohol, one part sport, one part dirt, stir gently: Beer commercials and television sports. In L.R. Vandeberg and L.A. Wenner (eds) *Television criticism: Approaches and applications.* New York: Longman, pp. 388–407.

Whannel, G. (1999) Sports stars, narrativization and masculinities. *Leisure Studies* 18(3): 249–65.

Wheaton, B. (2013) *The cultural politics of lifestyle sports.* London: Routledge.

Wheaton, B. (2009) The cultural politics of lifestyle sport (re)visited: Beyond white male lifestyles. In J. Ormond and B. Wheaton (eds) *'On the edge': Leisure, consumption and the representation of adventure sport* 104. Eastbourne: Leisure Studies Association, pp. 131–60.

Wheaton, B. (2003) Windsurfing: A subculture of commitment. In R. Rinehart and S. Sydor (eds) *To the extreme: Alternative sports, inside and out.* Albany, NY: State University of New York Press, pp. 75–101.

White, A. and Witty, K. (2009) Men's under use of health services – Finding alternative approaches. *Journal of Men's Health* 6(2): 95–7.

Williams, J., Dunning, E. and Murphy, P. (1989). *Hooligans abroad* (2nd edition). London: Routledge.

Williams, L. (2013) *Changing lives, changing drug journeys: Drug taking decisions from adolescence to adulthood.* London: Routledge.

Wilson, T.M. (2005) Drinking cultures: Sites and practices in the production and expression of identity. In T.M. Wilson (ed.) *Drinking Cultures: Alcohol and Identity.* Oxford and New York: Berg, pp. 1–24.

Winslow, S. and Hall, S. (2006) *Violent night: Urban leisure and contemporary culture.* London: Bloomsbury Academic.

Winter, I. (2000) Social capital and public policy in context. In Ian Winter (ed.) *Social capital and public policy in Australia.* Canberra: Australian Institute of Family Studies, Commonwealth of Australia, pp. 1–16.

World Health Organization (2011) *Global Health Risks. Mortality and Burden of Disease Attributable to Selected Major Risks.* Geneva, Switzerland: WHO.

Wyn, J. (2009) *Youth Health and Welfare: The Cultural Politics of Education and Wellbeing.* Melbourne: Oxford University Press.

Young, K., White, P. and McTeer, W. (1994) Body Talk: Male Athletes Reflect on Sport, injury and Pain. *Journal of Sport and Social Issues* 11: 175–94.

Young, M. (1995). Getting legless, falling down pissy arsed drunk: Policing men's leisure. *Journal of Gender Studies* 4(1).

Yu, J. and Bairner, A. (2012) Confucianism, baseball and ethnic stereotyping in Taiwan. *International Review for the Sociology of Sport* 47(6): 690–704.

Zajdow, G. (2010) It blasted me into space: intoxication and an ethics of pleasure. *Health sociology review* 19(2): 218–22.

Index

For Product Safety Concerns and Information please contact our EU
representative GPSR@taylorandfrancis.com
Taylor & Francis Verlag GmbH, Kaufingerstraße 24, 80331 München, Germany